THE
WOMAN WHO
SWALLOWED
A TOOTHBRUSH
and Other Bizarre Medical Cases

Copyright © Rob Myers, 2003

Published by ECW PRESS
2120 Queen Street East, Suite 200, Toronto, Ontario, Canada M4E 1E2

NATIONAL LIBRARY OF CANADA CATALOGUING IN PUBLICATION DATA

Myers, Rob
The woman who swallowed a toothbrush and other bizarre medical cases/ Rob Myers.
ISBN 1-55022-569-3

1. Medicine — Miscellanea.   2. Medicine — Anecdotes.   I. Title
RM706.M84 2002   610   C2002-905416-8

Editor: Tracey Millen
Cover and Text Design: Tania Craan
Typesetting: Wiesia Kolasinska
Production: Mary Bowness
Printing: Transcontinental
Cover images: Toothbrush©2003 Comstock Images,
X-ray©Tony Stone Imaging / Getty Images

This book is set in Minion and Trajan

The publication of *The Woman Who Swallowed a Toothbrush* has been generously
supported by the Canada Council, the Ontario Arts Council, and the
Government of Canada through the Book Publishing Industry
Development Program. **Canadä**

DISTRIBUTION

CANADA: Jaguar Book Group, 100 Armstrong Avenue, Georgetown, ON L7G 5S4

UNITED STATES: Independent Publishers Group, 814 North Franklin Street,
Chicago, Illinois 60610

EUROPE: Turnaround Publisher Services, Unit 3, Olympia Trading Estate,
Coburg Road, Wood Green, London N2Z 6T2

AUSTRALIA AND NEW ZEALAND: Wakefield Press, 1 The Parade West (Box 2266),
Kent Town, South Australia 5071

PRINTED AND BOUND IN CANADA

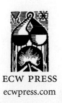

ECW PRESS
ecwpress.com

THE
WOMAN WHO
SWALLOWED
A TOOTHBRUSH
and Other Bizarre
Medical Cases

ROB MYERS, M.D.

ECW PRESS

To my wife Randi and my children Seth, Rachel, and Aaron

TABLE OF CONTENTS

INTRODUCTION

Most medicine is mundane. Clinical presentations fall into predictable patterns, which are rapidly recognized by the seasoned doctor. Some medical specialties are more interesting than others, but ultimately, when you've seen one you've usually seen them all. The adolescent belief that a gynecologist's job must be rewarding every moment of every day is not shared by most gynecologists. Those few who agree should probably be placed under surveillance.

This book documents some of the exceptional problems for which patients seek help. Every doctor has been involved in memorable medical cases. These stories are rare, at times profoundly tragic, even bordering on the unbelievable. Whereas 99.9% of medicine is predictable, this book is a sample of the other 0.1%.

I have always been interested in the world of the strange but true. Well-worn paperbacks from the *Ripley's Believe It or Not* series held an esteemed place in the drawer beside the toilet in the upstairs bathroom of the house in which I grew up. A full decade before graduating to *Playboy* magazine, I sat until my buttocks were numb reading *Ripley*.

Medical journals are similarly fascinating. I came across the story of a woman with a toothbrush lodged in her esophagus. After reading the conclusion to this bizarre tale, I decided to catalogue strange, documented tales of medical intrigue.

Though the names have been changed, the stories are real. One might question why any modification of these one-of-a-kind vignettes is necessary. The identifying data, even in its most skeletal form, is like DNA. The likelihood of these events affecting anyone else in the world should be one in a few billion.

And yet, after completing my research for the "Toothbrush" book, as my publisher and I call it, I found an account in the lay press of the same toothbrush scenario. I e-mailed the writer to suggest that an alternative explanation for the seemingly innocent act of toothbrush swallowing should be pursued with the young lady. Read on and you will soon discover why not all is as it seems in medicine.

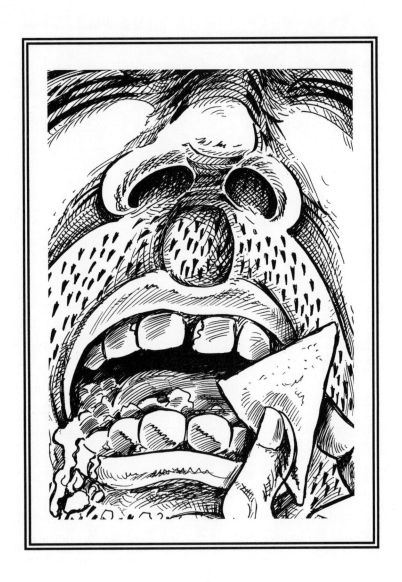

FULL

Emergency room doctors and nurses are in a constant state of languid preparedness. Periods of boredom are quickly replaced by life-threatening heart attacks, traumas, and other terrible conditions. Shards of broken bones poking through bloodied skin, slippery intestines protruding through bullet holes, severe head injuries — anything that can go wrong with the human body may result in an emergency room visit at any time, day or night.

On a quiet Wednesday evening approaching midnight, sirens wailed and lights flashed as a 56-year-old man arrived at the emergency department via ambulance. He had awoken from a restless sleep 30 minutes earlier with sudden severe abdominal pain. He quickly called 911. Though he lived close by, it took the two slender paramedics longer than expected to load his obese 5'6" 450-pound frame into the ambulance.

His folds spilled over the sides of a narrow hospital gurney in the triage room, as the skeletonized version of his story was elicited by the triage nurse. A quick check of his vital signs indicated that beyond his girth, there was a serious problem afoot.

He was tachycardic (had a rapid heart rate) with a pulse of 120 beats per minute. His blood pressure was low at 90/60, he was feverish and breathing rapidly. Oxygen, an intravenous line, and a cardiac monitor — all the basics — were in place as the emergency room physician appeared. The curtain rattled as he entered the tiny cubicle.

"What brings you to hospital Mr. Canderas?" he inquired.

"I don't feel so good" was the unhelpful reply.

"Could you be more specific?" the doctor continued.

"Well, I couldn't get to sleep so I got out of bed around 10 p.m. and fixed myself a snack and watched some TV." It seemed to take a huge effort to speak.

The doctor couldn't imagine that the large man before him could walk or fix a snack. "Must sleep in the kitchen," he thought.

"I must have dozed off in the chair," the patient

continued. "I carried myself over to bed and lay down but I didn't feel right, sort of like I ate too much."

"Go on, go on," said the doctor.

"I suddenly got this horrible stomach pain. I puked all over the bed and called an ambulance."

The doctor moved over to the middle of the bed and worked on Mr. Canderas's abdomen. His hands were lost, enveloped by moist pockets and crevasses, surrounded by smooth waves of rubbery tissue. He watched Mr. Canderas's face as he poked and prodded his abdomen. Then it came. Not a subtle grimace of displeasure, but a yelp so painful and piteous that were he 300 pounds lighter, parts of him surely would have jumped off the bed.

Diving through fat, the doctor's hands had landed on a rigid board-like abdomen. Irritation within the peritoneal cavity, as with appendicitis or liver injury, causes severe pain with rigidity of the abdominal muscles. This man had an acute abdomen. With the associated fever, fast heart rate (tachycardia), and relatively low blood pressure (hypotension), an emergency surgical exploration (laparotomy) was necessary.

The wheeled gurney squeaked and strained under the weight as Mr. Canderas was transported to the operating room, where the centerpiece is the surgical table (although surgeons may disagree). Surgical tables are standard issue and, consequently, narrow. This presented a problem for Mr. Canderas, as the table could accommodate perhaps one of his fleshy limbs. A fleet of four tables and half a dozen of the O.R. night staff was required to finally secure nearly a quarter ton of limp tissue and ready it for the knife.

He was anesthetized and intubated. The surgeon sliced and sliced and sliced. Yellow flecks of fat melted and dripped into the surgical field, lit by a blazing overhead light. Pools of blood formed and were quickly drained by a suction catheter. The peritoneal lining appeared like a thick piece of Saran wrap, embedded with a criss-cross of minute blood vessels. The scalpel rose and fell, and there was silence, punctuated by the staccato beep of the heart rate monitor.

Doritos. It was not initially clear whether they were cheese flavored or spicy, but they were definitely Doritos, caked in what looked like cake. A corner of a Pop-tart, the size of a quarter, slipped out, fighting with the Doritos for release from the confines of the abdominal cavity. What in the world were undigested, and in many respects unchewed, food particles doing swimming about Mr. Canderas's abdominal cavity? How did they get out of the stomach and gastrointestinal tract?

A visual inspection of the stomach secured the diagnosis: a linear tear along the lesser curvature of the stomach, like a crevasse in a mountain. His stomach had quite simply burst. Excessive ingestion of food and drink was more than his stomach could handle. Fill up the tank and the gas will spill out. Fill up the stomach and vomit, or it will rupture.

Mr. Canderas spent two weeks in the ICU, ventilated on a respirator. Antibiotics were poured into his bloodstream around the clock, carried off to fight the infection in his abdomen. He finally turned the corner and gradually improved. After a month-long hospital stay he was ready for discharge, 93 pounds lighter. The advice from his physicians was simple: don't eat when you're full.

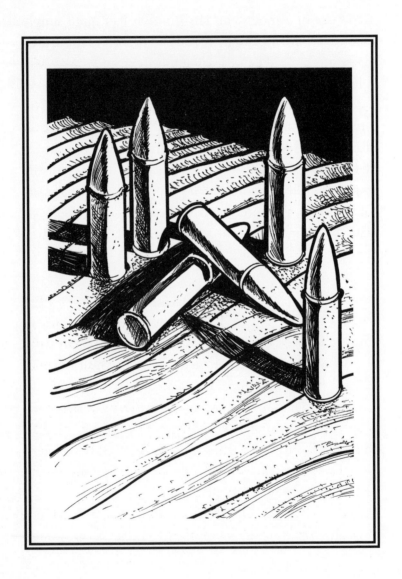

BULLET

An Iranian man was admitted to the orthopedic ward for elective back surgery. Orthopedic surgeons are renowned for their impressive surgical skills. They are excellent with a hammer and nail, but many are less adept at histories and physical examination.

Notwithstanding, the orthopedic resident mustered all of his exam skills and placed his stethoscope in the "tripod" position. The tripod position is just below the sternum. This placement allows a surgeon to listen to the heart, lungs, and abdomen at the same time.

"What's this?" he thought. "I hear something." A sound whooshed through the stethoscope tubing to the young trainee's ears. It was loud and it was obvious. You didn't need a medical degree to know that this was an abnormal sound.

The orthopod thought the murmur was too loud to be a normal variant, though had no idea what the origin could be, so he postponed surgery and sent the man for an echocardiogram. Echos utilize ultrasound waves to image the heart, akin to ultrasound technology that examines the fetus of a pregnant woman. Abnormal heart sounds, like murmurs, may be benign, or reflect serious cardiac disease.

The patient spoke no English, and a Farsee interpreter was unavailable. Through a mixture of hand signals and cajoling, the man was directed to lie on his left side as the technologist took the microphone-shaped probe and placed it on the man's chest.

As the cardiac anatomy was uncovered, the technologist saw an uncommon though not unusual abnormality. The young Iranian had a small hole in his heart known as a ventricular septal defect (VSD). VSDs are a type of shunt, an abnormal communication between two parts of the heart. The abnormality may cause excess blood flow into the wrong chamber of the heart.

As the probe glided across the gel-smeared chest, another oddity appeared. "What was sitting in the apex of the left ventricle?" thought the technologist. The left ventricle is the heart's largest and strongest chamber, while the apex is the lowermost portion. Embedded in the patient's heart was a bright oblong object. Clearly this was neither a tumor nor a blood clot. She was at a loss. Despite 20 years of experience and thousands of echocardiograms, she had never seen anything like this. And what did it have to do with the vsd, if anything? She called the cardiologist.

He too was baffled. Other than a tumor or blood clot, he could think of no other possibility, and yet it looked like neither. "Let's get a chest x-ray," he said. "Maybe that will help."

An hour later he had the chest x-ray in his hands, and secured it on the x-ray viewer, an illuminating light source. "The object is shaped like a bullet," he said. He went back to the patient and examined his chest. A small two-inch scar was present just below his breastbone (sternum). With the aid of an interpreter, he was able to piece together the story.

While patrolling the Iran-Iraq border during the war of the 1980s, the patient encountered a platoon of Iraqi soldiers attempting a cross-border infiltration. Shots were exchanged, and the young Iranian fell to the dust, blood pouring from his chest. A makeshift stretcher was fashioned and after an agonizing wait on the battlefield, he was rushed to a military hospital. He remained for three weeks of observation, and was discharged with little information about his condition, save for a warning that his heart was damaged. He felt well, with no cardiac and respiratory symptoms. The murmur had gone undetected on his immigration physical exam.

A CAT scan of his chest confirmed the story. A bullet pierced his chest, ricocheted off a rib, crossed the ventricles of his heart (causing a VSD), and, slowed by its journey, embedded itself into the apex of his left ventricle. This was the first reported case of a bullet causing a VSD, staying in the heart, and causing no symptoms. As there appeared to be no hemodynamic compromise, no symptoms, and no other adverse affects on the heart, no surgery was advised, and he was subsequently lost to follow-up.

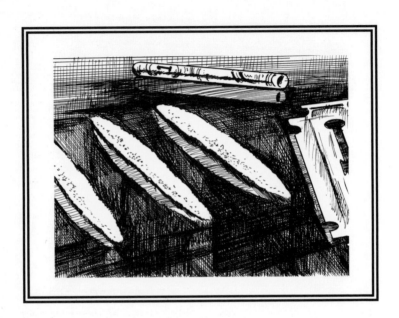

BEWARE OF MINERAL OIL

A young woman of 25 presented to the hospital after collapsing on an airplane. She was traveling from Ecuador to her home in New York City. In the middle of the flight she suddenly stood up, clumsily bolted forward, and tripped over other passengers onto the carpeted aisle. She cried out in anguish as she keeled over. A physician (a pathologist unfortunately) was on the same flight, but could offer little help except for an autopsy were it necessary. He recalled enough medical training to turn her on her side to prevent her from aspirating her lunch, a portion of which she had just emptied from her stomach.

She was taken to the back of the plane and laid across three seats. She was screaming and kicking and required restraints. The pilot decided to divert the airplane to Dallas.

Over the following 15 minutes her abdominal pain became progressively intense. Her behavior was increasingly bizarre and erratic. "I must get to the washroom!" she yelled.

A kind elderly woman, certain this was simply a case of psychotic constipation, offered the woman her mineral oil. "A laxative will help dear, just take this," she said.

The woman was in and out of consciousness. By the time the plane landed and taxied toward the gate, her condition had deteriorated. She was lifted into the ambulance and driven to hospital.

In the emergency room, restraints secured her to the stretcher. Her main complaint was severe abdominal pain. Yelling in a mixture of English and Spanish, she was hallucinating and perspiring heavily. She screamed at the unseen spiders under her skin, and prayed to a hovering angel. On exam, her heart rate was racing at 160 beats per minute, and her blood pressure was dangerously elevated at 250/130. Her pupils were dilated, her skin gray. She resembled Linda Blair from the movie *The Exorcist*. Her abdomen was exquisitely tender and board-like. This was a surgical emergency. A ruptured appendix? A tubal pregnancy? A bad meal the night before?

The surgeon was called. He was new to the hospital, in his first year after a decade of training and sleeplessness. Miss Ecuador was sped to the operating room, kicking and screaming against the binds on her wrists and ankles, spewing a stream of incomprehensible insults, spinning her vomit-riddled hair wildly.

A 500-watt beam of light shone on the surgical field from an overhead lamp. The patient's smooth skin was cut from navel to sternum. A shallow river of blood formed and fell down the sides of her abdomen. The surgeon stared inside the cave he had cut.

"Nothing wrong on a surface inspection of the intra-abdominal contents," the doctor noted.

His size 7½ gloved hands entered the abdomen and explored, desperately searching for the problem. Suddenly they grabbed it like a football. It was her stomach, over-grown and distended to twice its normal size. Through the translucent mucosa of her intestinal walls he caught a terrifying sight. Long cylindrical tubes, like enormous fly larvae, were infesting her intestines and presumably her stomach. He let out a gasp, shocked at what he was witnessing. With trembling hands he cut into her stomach, prepared to leap backwards and save himself. Sweat stained his back and chest. What ghoulish form would fly forward when released from the confines of the stomach?

Condoms spilled out. Dozens and dozens of condoms, each filled with a fortune in cocaine. The lass from Quito was a body-packer. Surgical buckets, often used for entrails, a transplanted organ, or other body parts were filled one after the other with condom packages of cocaine. Five buckets overflowed with 178 condoms, 45 of which were ruptured.

As the surgeon was transferring the horde, the patient suffered a sudden cardiac arrest. Despite massive and prolonged resuscitation efforts, she died on the operating room table. The diagnosis, confirmed with post-mortem blood analysis, was acute cocaine intoxication.

Each of the 178 condoms contained approximately 4.5 grams of cocaine, for a total of 800 grams (nearly a kilo). Depending upon the frequency of recreational use, and thus tolerance to its effects, a lethal dosage of cocaine is approximately two grams. This young woman had ingested 400 times that amount.

The burden of so many packages had distended her stomach and intestines, causing severe abdominal pain. Perhaps one had ruptured, releasing a stream of cocaine into her body. Unfortunately, the mineral oil acted upon the latex of the condoms, and dissolved them. By mistakenly offering a mineral oil cocktail, the elderly woman inadvertently contributed to the demise of the patient. The mineral oil caused the release of toxic amounts of cocaine, resulting in cardiovascular collapse and death.

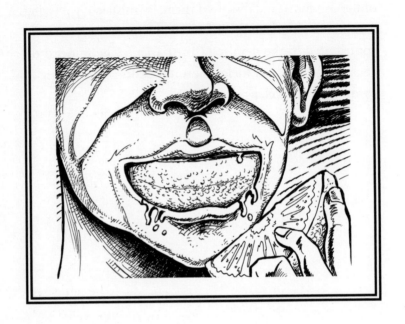

SWOLLEN GUMS

A seven-year-old boy was taken to the pediatrician complaining of leg pain and swollen, bleeding gums. His height and weight were average. He had been developing normally and had never been hospitalized. He was a healthy and energetic boy until his symptoms began two months previously.

His appetite was poor and he was peevish and irritable. He had developed mild diarrhea. His leg pain had become suddenly unbearable that day, but he soldiered on and walked into the examining room with a grimace. On exam, both weight and height had slipped considerably over the year. There was a mild fever. His gums were swollen and blue, bleeding easily when touched. Little red spots had erupted all over his skin, as if he had been pricked by thousands of tiny needles. Miniature droplets of blood oozed from his hair follicles.

Fearing a severe illness, the pediatrician immediately admitted the boy to hospital. He underwent numerous investigations over the following week. Blood tests showed a low red blood cell count, consistent with mild anemia. X-rays showed abnormally thin bones. Leukemia was considered, but an examination of his bone marrow showed no abnormal cells. He was poked everywhere. Blood was sent to biochemistry, hematology, microbiology, and pathology, but still there was no clear diagnosis for his puzzling condition.

The pediatrician, trained in North America, was dumbfounded. What in the world was going on? He sought assistance from his colleagues, and not one could provide insight. He decided to present the case to a large pediatric group during weekly diagnostic rounds.

An elderly doctor, retired for a decade, enjoyed attending these rounds. He had completed medical school and pediatrics in India. His passion for medicine remained as strong as it had been 60 years ago, when he graduated from medical school in Madras. Though he had leg pain, related to age and arthritis, every Friday morning he arose early, put on his faded brown suit and wide striped tie, slicked back his thin white hair and rode the subway downtown.

The conference room was always full. The hospital pediatricians sat at the front, perched in their thrones, supremely confident in their skills. The trainees sat behind the staff, respecting the hierarchy of their respective positions. The retired pediatrician always occupied the back row. Punctual, he shuffled with his cane and sat down quietly, unnoticed by those around him. The lights were dimmed and the case was presented to the group. Slides of the boy's results were flashed on the screen. They showed his blood, they showed his bones, they even showed the boy. A great debate ensued. Diagnoses were strewn about and discarded.

"Have you considered Histiocytosis? Blastomycosis? Mastocytosis?" "Could it be rheumatic fever, poliomyelitis, or septic arthritis?" "What about syphilis or osteomyelitis?"

The elderly pediatrician recognized the diagnosis an hour previously, only minutes into the presentation. He raised his hand. No one noticed. He stood up. No response. He cleared his throat. Still nothing. The hour was up. The room remained baffled.

"Any other comments?" asked the boy's pediatrician, dejected and defeated by the failure of the group to help. As they began to depart, he pointed to an elderly gentleman in the back.

His frail voice carried forward to the front of the lecture theater. "He has scurvy."

Scurvy. Vitamin C deficiency. The boy had scurvy. Having seen hundreds of cases in India, it was as easy as a cold to diagnose. The room was silent and embarrassed, for they knew he was right. They had missed a simple case of scurvy. He turned and left, shuffling back to the subway.

A detailed dietary history was obtained, having been neglected on admission. The boy's diet consisted exclusively of cookies, bread, yogurt, and milk for nearly a year — no vegetables, no fruit, and no meat. His mother felt he would naturally return to a more balanced diet in time. The habit had become a dietary obsession.

He was treated with 300 milligrams of ascorbic acid (Vitamin C). Within one week he was asymptomatic and normal. A dietitian was consulted to educate the parents and child.

The first clinical descriptions of scurvy were recorded in Egypt 3,500 years ago. Scurvy was a frequent problem for sailors in the 18th century. In 1746, James Lind, a British doctor, discovered that citrus fruits cured the disease. He may not have understood why, but the empiric cure was effective nonetheless. British sailors were given lemon and lime juice (thus the term limeys) on subsequent voyages.

Vitamin C deficiency impairs collagen synthesis.

Collagen is an important building block of bone and tissues, and its absence leads to weakness in the body's architecture, impairing bone and teeth development and causing bleeding.

Scurvy is rare in North America, and more common in impoverished Third World countries.

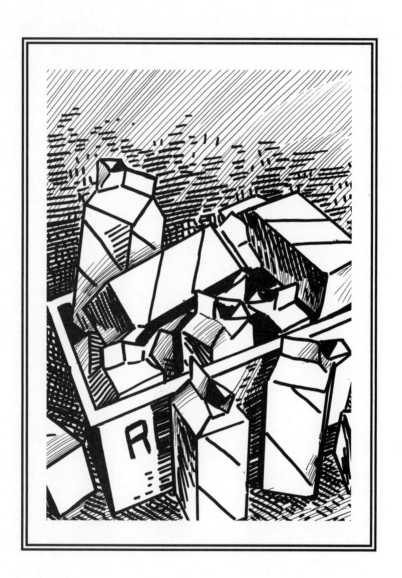

NEAR DEATH BY POTASSIUM

A 48-year-old woman was admitted to hospital with fatigue and a poor appetite over the preceding week. Her history was unremarkable. She had no previous illnesses and was on no medications. The physical examination was non-contributory. As part of routine emergency room procedures, a few vials of blood were sent to the biochemistry and hematology labs. Thirty minutes later, a phone call was made from the biochemistry lab to the emergency room doctor. "Mrs. Stevens has a potassium level of 8.2 mmol/L. I've checked it three times."

A normal potassium level is 3.5–5.0 mmol/L. A potassium of eight is critical, and immediately life-threatening.

It is associated with severe cardiac rhythm disturbances, and may cause rapid death if untreated.

The doctor sprang to his feet, barking orders to the nurse. "Get bed six into the acute room now, her potassium is over eight. I need a stat ECG." Mrs. Stevens was rushed into the acute room and bundled onto a waiting stretcher. An intravenous was deftly placed into her arm and connected to a bag of saline. An oxygen mask was thrust onto her face.

"One amp of IV calcium stat." The doctor's voice was calm and clear. "And I want IV insulin and an amp of D50W. Let's get 50 cc of Kayxelate and 50 cc of sorbitol orally now." Nurses buzzed about, and within minutes tubes were filled and liquids administered. Definitive treatment was underway.

There are few causes of hyperkalemia (high potassium) of such severity, and all are easily diagnosed. Either you are taking in too much or the kidneys can't get rid of normal amounts. The emergency room physician went to work, mentally checking off the causes as he excluded them one by one.

One of the most common causes of hyperkalemia is renal failure, acute or chronic. The kidneys are filters, ridding the body of numerous waste products, and are important regulators of the body's potassium. Renal impairment, characterized by a rise in serum creatinine, causes hyperkalemia. Mrs. Stevens's kidney function was normal.

"One down," he thought.

At times, if blood is drawn through the needle too vigorously, red blood cells break apart in a process called hemolysis. Hemolysis releases potassium from the blood cells into the serum component, resulting in a falsely elevated reading. The lab had checked the specimen three times, and no hemolysis was detected. Two down.

Some medications, including potassium supplements, raise serum potassium. The physician again checked with Mrs. Stevens. She was taking no pills, either prescribed or herbal. Three down. Further tests were ordered, blood was squeezed from her body, yet no cause was identified. Within days, her potassium normalized, and the doctors scratched their heads.

An enterprising intern, with a quality for attention to detail found only in newly ordained doctors, returned to the bedside of Mrs. Stevens to review her story. After 30 fruitless minutes he prepared to leave.

"What about orange juice?" she asked. "Could that have anything to do with this?"

His ears perked up, and he turned to face her. "Only if

you were drinking liters," he said. "Are you?" She looked sheepish. "Kind of," came her response.

She was a willing participant in *The Orange Juice Diet*. A health food store in her neighborhood trumpeted the benefits of organic orange juice (purchased in their store of course) to "cure hidden disease and lose unwanted fat." Mrs. Stevens had been drinking 5 liters of orange juice per day for three months. She had unintentionally intoxicated herself with liters of potassium rich orange juice. Simple dietary modification prevented further life-threatening emergencies.

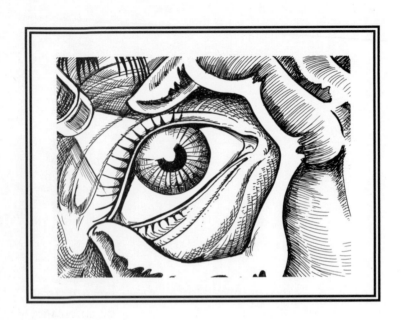

LAZARUS
PHENOMENON

A 22-year-old, apparently a frequent user of illicit drugs, was brought to the emergency room at 3 a.m. by ambulance VSA (vital signs absent). He was found unconscious in the middle of the dance floor of an all-night club. Witnesses said he had been dancing wildly for hours and suddenly collapsed onto the floor. The paramedics waded through the crowd of drugged-out teenagers and young adults in the darkened club, with flashes of bright colored lights streaming across the floor.

Not much space had been cleared by the patrons, who seemed unaware of the unfolding drama. The man was motionless. His breathing came in short shallow gasps, and his lips were blue. The paramedics quickly intubated him, in the middle of the dance floor, observed by only a few drunken stuporous kids.

A clear curved plastic tube (an endotracheal tube) was impaled into his throat, forcibly opened by a steel laryngoscope. The tube split his vocal cords and settled just above the lungs. An air bag was quickly attached and his lungs were manually inflated by one of the paramedics. An intravenous was inserted into an arm fresh with needle marks, and a monitor was attached to his chest. No pulse was found. The electrical blips on the monitor screen showed erratic meaningless twists. He was in ventricular fibrillation, a fatal rhythm that produces no cardiac output. Unless normal rhythm is restored within minutes, brain death or worse ensues.

Two rectangular paddles, attached to the monitor by long cords, were quickly placed on the boy's chest. "360 joules. Clear!" yelled the paramedic. A jolt of electricity shot through the boy. His body jerked upwards spasmodically, as if raised from the dead, then fell to the dance floor, motionless. The monitor showed v.fib again. "Again. Stay at 360. Clear," repeated the medic.

Five times they shocked him and five times he remained pulseless. A bolus of amiodarone was shot into his vein. Cardiopulmonary resuscitation (CPR) continued. The paramedics took turns pumping his chest and squeezing air into his lungs. All the while, colored lights flashed in the club. Patrons were murmuring. The night was still young and they wanted to party. Small white flashes, party tablets, could be seen passing between desperate hands.

The paramedics rushed the boy to the ambulance, a path cleared by burly tattooed bouncers, and the party continued.

In the emergency department, the boy looked dead. He was asystolic, his heart was not generating any electrical activity, and he had no spontaneous breathing. He was lifeless, but he was young. Doctors never give up too early in the young. Drug after drug was infused. Epinephrine, naloxone, atropine, lidocaine, bicarb, amiodarone, bretylium. Hands pumped on his chest, external hearts forcing blood around his circuitry. All the while the respirator breathed for him, pushing 100% oxygen into his lungs.

Despite these Herculean efforts, nothing changed. His heart had stopped, and would not respond to the flogging. They were working on a dead man. A casualty of the excesses of youth. Ecstasy. Heroin. It didn't matter. The emergency team leader called the arrest to a halt 82 minutes after arrival. He was declared dead. The tubes were left in place, customary for a coroner's case. The doctors and nurses moved on to the living.

Within two minutes, the emergency physician was

summoned with a loud cry. The nurse was preparing the body when the monitor suddenly showed an electrical rhythm. A blood pressure of 90/60 was also recorded. Shocked medical staff returned and initiated new treatment protocols. The boy was hooked up to a ventilator and transferred to the critical care unit.

He remained in the ICU for two months, fighting complications such as sepsis, pneumonia, and kidney failure. After three months in hospital, he was discharged home with no evidence of neurologic impairment. He had lived — it was a miracle. The boy was one of a few reported cases of the Lazarus phenomenon.

The term Lazarus phenomenon was first coined in 1982, to describe the unexpected return of circulation and breathing after declaration of death. Less than 30 cases have been reported in the medical literature. There is no single explanation for the miracle of the Lazarus phenomenon.

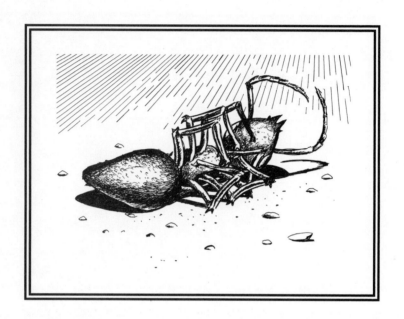

EARWIGS AND MOSQUITOES

A 40-year-old South African was visiting Namibia during a one-day stopover en route to the United States. He was an important religious figure, and was traveling during the apartheid era to gain support for political change in his country.

Shortly after arriving at his hotel in Namibia, he complained of nausea, vomiting, diarrhea, abdominal pain, and weakness. He was admitted to hospital. Though his symptoms were profound and sudden at their onset, they quickly resolved and he was discharged the following day after adequate intravenous rehydration, with a provisional diagnosis of stomach flu or food poisoning. He resumed his journey.

Upon his arrival in the U.S.A., he checked into his room at the Marriott. His symptoms returned suddenly and ferociously. Abdominal pain, nausea, vomiting, and diarrhea attacked him. He was overcome with weakness, and barely found the strength to dial the ambulance number. The paramedics found him lying on the carpet beside the bed. He was diaphoretic (sweaty) and his muscles twitched uncontrollably. After a quick check, they transported him to the hospital, sirens screaming.

His amylase level, a marker of an inflamed pancreas, was elevated. Yet his recovery was rapid and complete, with his amylase returning to normal. He was again discharged, this time with a diagnosis of pancreatitis. He returned to the hotel.

He was re-admitted within 24 hours with confusion and anxiety. He was hyperventilating and his blood phosphate level was low. His abdominal symptoms had returned. He was diagnosed with post-traumatic stress syndrome by confused medical staff, and, for the third time, discharged from hospital.

He returned to his hotel. While preparing for a political dinner meeting, he was overcome with nausea and abdominal pain. He was admitted to hospital for the fourth time. He was salivating copiously, and sweating through his clothes. His eyes roamed uncontrollably. He could not walk straight and had the appearance of a drunkard. He vomited, had diarrhea, and lost control of his bladder. Fluid was coming from everywhere.

An astute emergency room doctor, the son of a farmer, recognized the diverse constellation of symptoms. He had seen this before when a farm worker was accidentally exposed to insecticide. This man was suffering from acute organophosphate (an insecticide) poisoning.

The diagnosis was confirmed with specific blood tests. No active treatment was indicated. He was discharged and told to discard not only his clothes, but his suitcase as well. It was suspected, and later confirmed, that the contents of his luggage had been intentionally contaminated with organophosphate poison prior to his departure for Namibia. He had been the victim of an attempted assassination.

Years later, after ascending the government ladder in the post-apartheid era, he was employed as a policy maker in the new administration. An inquiry into the covert practices of the apartheid regime was organized under his jurisdiction. The inquiry discovered that a special South

African military unit, an extension of the South African Civil Corporation Bureau, had killed hundreds of apartheid activists by poisoning.

The man's clothes had been covered in organophosphate, and each time he returned to his hotel room, the dust was absorbed through his skin, causing acute poisoning. While in hospital, he was dressed in a sterile gown, and thus quickly recovered. He is the only known survivor of organophosphate warfare.

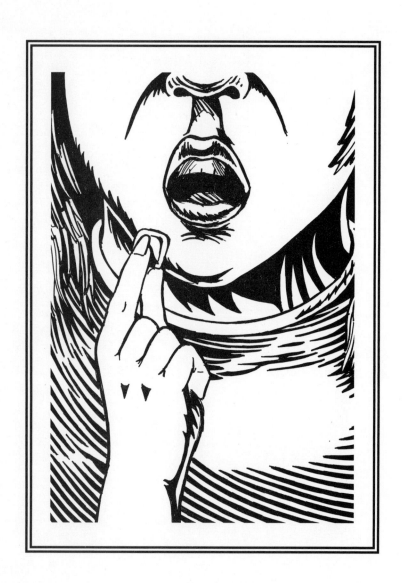

AIRPLANE
LAVATORY

An airline stewardess, Ms. Fitzhenry, presented to her family
physician with a seven-year history of frequent daily diarrhea and abdominal cramps.

A young woman of 26, she was frequently ribbed by her
colleagues for using the airplane lavatory more often than
all of the passengers combined. After numerous outpatient
investigations yielded no clue to the origin of her symptoms, she was electively admitted to the gastrointestinal
unit of a teaching hospital for further tests.

Her abdominal pain was around her navel (called peri-
umbilical). Its onset heralded explosive diarrhea. She had
up to a dozen watery, small volume, light brown, gas-filled

bowel movements per day. Otherwise healthy, she had had an appendectomy as a child. Her only medication was oral contraception. Her HIV test was negative, other blood tests were unremarkable, and an abdominal ultrasound and abdominal CAT scan were both normal.

A pleasant little test, called a colonoscopy, was arranged. A very long, flexible tube is lubricated and gently inserted into the anus as far as it will go. In preparation for the test, the bowels must be devoid of stool. This is accomplished with four liters of a sweet-tasting liquid called "GoLytely," an absolute misnomer. GoLytely flushes out the bowel in multiple cascades of liquid stool. It makes one wonder what drives gastroenterologists to practice their specialty. Patients are sedated, an obvious necessity when yards of tubing are guided through yards of bowels.

The colonoscope has a camera system allowing direct visualization of the bowel walls from the inside. This explains why stool is cleared away beforehand. If the bowels are misshapen, inflamed, or growing polyps or tumors, the colonoscope will diagnose the problem. It also comes with a nifty device called alligator forceps, which allow the doctor to sample a piece of bowel for study in the lab.

With gritted teeth the stewardess consented to the procedure.

Not a scratch or mark was identified on her beautiful translucent colon, and the biopsy specimen confirmed her bowel was normal.

A good doctor, like a good detective, practices the art of sleuthing. An expert specialist knows all of the causes of all of the symptoms encompassed by his or her specialty. Common things top the list, which is mentally checked as stories unfold and physical examinations are performed. Along the way, tests are used in a logical sequence, to either rule in or exclude a suspected diagnosis. Ms. Fitzhenry's problem was getting further and further down the list. Numerous standard investigations had turned up no cause for her copious stools.

The doctors considered laxative abuse, an occasional practice of young slender women and the cause of up to 15% of chronic diarrhea. A urinalysis, which can identify traces of laxatives, was negative.

Her stool was collected daily for three days and weighed. The nurses were not paid time and a half to collect the specimens. The normal weight of stools over 24 hours is less than 250 grams. Ms. Fitzhenry's "collection" weighed three times more. What was weighing down her stools, causing such massive diarrhea?

An intravenous was inserted and she was asked to fast for 24 hours. During the study period her diarrhea resolved completely. This was diagnostic of "osmotic diarrhea." Diarrhea may be osmotic or secretory. A secretory diarrhea, caused by any of a multitude of intestinal diseases, does not respond to fasting. There was no need to continue down the checklist.

Osmotic diarrhea implies the ingestion of an agent that is not absorbed through the intestines into the body, like GoLytely. It moves through the bowels like a cascade of water, taking with it all of the contents until it all comes out the chute in the end, as diarrhea.

What was she hiding? What was she eating? Why was she eating it?

As it turned out, she was hiding nothing. With a more detailed history, it was innocently offered by Ms. Fitzhenry that she chewed up to 60 sticks of sugarless gum a day and had been doing so for seven years. Each stick of gum contained 1.25 grams of sorbitol, a non-absorbable, non-digestible osmotic agent. She was ingesting 75 grams daily. Doses as small as 10 grams may cause diarrhea. She was an unintentional laxative abuser.

She stopped chewing the gum, which was cathartic because as soon as she stopped, her bowel habits returned to normal.

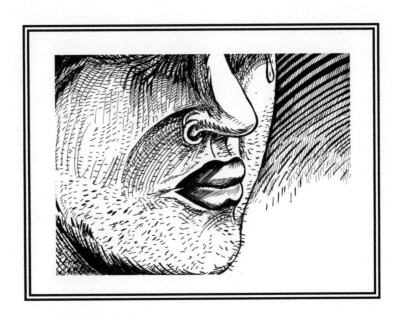

HOT FLASHES
IN A MAN

A 42-year-old man was seen by his doctor complaining of hot flashes and swollen, tender breast tissue (gynecomastia). A quick check confirmed he was as advertised, anatomically male. The general practitioner had a busy practice, churning through 50–60 patients per day. He had no time to work up the problem, and no desire to see it through. He referred the patient to an endocrinologist for further evaluation.

David was an idiosyncratic character, with nipple rings, tongue piercings, and colorful tattoos decorating his chest, back, and arms. Single, he had no children and was employed as an accountant for a large computer software company. He admitted to occasional recreational drug use including ecstasy and marijuana, and denied cocaine or heroin abuse. He was on no prescribed or herbal medications and had no relevant past medical history. His exam disclosed normal male genitalia, hair where it should be, and unmistakable breasts, small for a woman but large for a man.

Four months later, after a series of investigations, he sat down with the endocrinologist. His doctor studied the blood test results carefully as the patient sat in the next room on the exam table, twiddling his thumbs and playing with his rings. David was wearing one of those flimsy hospital gowns. It was a blue cotton smock, open in the back and knee-high. He wore white sports socks, with blue and yellow stripes at the top.

"Mr. Jenkins," said the doctor. "I've reviewed your blood results and there are a number of problems we need to discuss."

The patient shifted uncomfortably, his bare buttocks sticking to the paper covering of his perch.

"Your testosterone levels are low," the doctor continued, "and your FSH and LH levels are elevated. Your growth hormone, prolactin, and some other hormone levels all rise appropriately with stimulation. Your serum cortisol and HCG are raised and your CAT scan showed normal adrenals and no intra-abdominal pathology."

"Speak English, Doc," came the reply.

"OK, let me put it this way. Your blood estrogen levels are high, which explains hot flashes and breast development. The question is where the estrogen is coming from. I have studied your blood and imaged your body. I can't find a source, and thought you might be able to help out. Are you taking female hormones?" he asked innocently but knowingly.

"Must be the urine," David replied.

As a child, David wasn't so sure he wanted to be a mister. He loved cross-dressing in private and public. Though heterosexual, he continued varying his gender identity.

Beginning five years earlier, he developed an unusual habit. As often as he could find a source, usually four or five times a week, he drank large amounts of female urine. His "source" was sexual partners, live-in girlfriends, or women he had met who wanted a few extra bucks. His interest became habit forming. Many of the women were taking some form of hormone supplementation, thus exposing him to large amounts of estrogen. He simply felt better, and didn't mind breast development.

Drinking one's own urine is a bizarre ancient practice popular in India. There is no scientific validity to the assertion that imbibing one's own liquid (or solid) waste is in some way cathartic or cleansing. Drinking the urine of others is just as remote in the annals of obscure medical cases. Mr. Jenkins made no apology, and simply requested that his physicians accept him as he was. Within years he suffered a heart attack, a known complication of excessive estrogen supplementation. His smoking surely didn't help. He continued smoking and "drinking" and was lost to further follow-up.

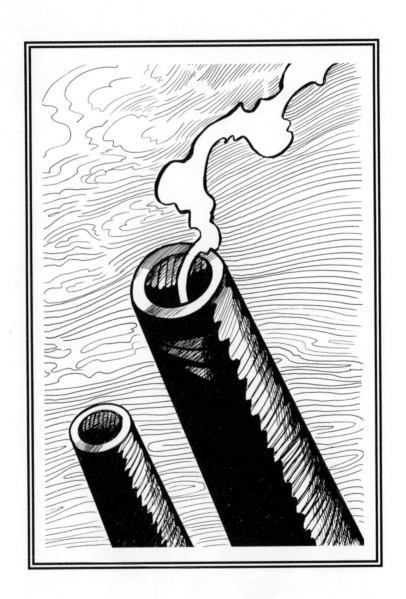

WINE BY
THE BARREL

A French soldier, celebrating initiation into an artillery regiment, drank a small quantity of wine during a party, had a grand-mal seizure, and collapsed into a coma. Others had partaken in the same ritual, but hastily vomited after drinking the cheap French Bordeaux. Corporal Château was rushed to hospital by his colleagues.

As was customary of his regiment, 250 ml. of wine was poured down the barrel of a 155 mm gun after shots were fired from it. Shortly after fulfilling the custom, he fell down shaking violently. "C'est une crise d'épilepsie, sacrebleu," cried his brethren.

He was carried on a stretcher raised above the heads of

six soldiers wearing gold metallic helmets and green army fatigues. They poured him into a military jeep and dropped him off at the emergency room entrance. Shaking violently, the young recruit's head was draped to the side. His eyes were open and unfocused. "Another drunken soldier," said the emergency room doctor (in French). "Give 15 milligrams of valium IM (intramuscular) now," he barked.

The seizures slowed and then disappeared. His military fatigues were removed and he was examined. His blood pressure and heart rate were fine, but he was completely unresponsive to verbal and physical stimulation. "Perhaps too much valium, n'est-ce pas?" said the doctor.

To evaluate neurologic activity, doctors will often squeeze the hell out of a finger or toe, or violently rub on the sternum, a stimulus that would evoke howls of displeasure in all but the brain dead.

Corporal Château was oblivious. The doctor was concerned about airway protection, worried the young man would choke on his vomit in such a stuporous state. He was thus hooked up to a ventilator after a tube was inserted into his lungs.

Now what? Blood tests were sent including an alcohol level. It came back at just above the legal limit for driving. This boy was in no shape to be a passenger. Alcohol poisoning was not the explanation for this presentation. There was also no blood or urine evidence of drug use such as cocaine or heroin. An MRI (magnetic resonance imaging) of his brain showed no bleeding or other abnormalities.

A lumbar puncture was performed, and the fluid was sent for analysis. The brain and spinal cord are bathed in about 150 ml. of a watery looking fluid called CSF (cerebrospinal fluid). Brain infections or bleeding can be detected by sampling this fluid, which is done by sticking a long skinny needle between the lower lumbar vertebrae in the back (thus the term lumbar puncture). The soldier was comatose and needed no sedation. The fluid analysis came back unremarkable. There was no sign of infection.

The physicians involved in the young man's care speculated about the role of the gun barrel. Blood and urine samples were sent for cyanide, mercury, and lead poisoning. They all came back negative.

Meanwhile, over the ensuing two days, while in the ICU, the soldier stopped producing urine and went into renal failure. Hemodialysis was initiated. It was an unusual sight; his bed was constantly swarmed by uniformed soldiers from his regiment, who provided a 24-hour vigil.

A fancy, rarely used test was employed, called inductively coupled plasma emission spectometry. It was suggested by one of the engineers from his regiment, in hopes of finding some otherwise unrecognized toxicity. It accomplished exactly that.

High concentrations of tungsten, a heavy metal, were detected in all fluid samples. His blood contained 2,000 times the usual measured concentration of tungsten detectable in humans. Tungsten is excreted by the kidneys. His urine had more than 200 times the expected amount.

Three days later, he suddenly regained consciousness, with no recollection of the events leading to his hospital admission. A kidney biopsy showed damage, probably due to the tungsten. There was, however, no precedent in the medical literature to confirm his renal failure was from tungsten poisoning.

Within two weeks his kidney function returned, and five weeks after admission he was discharged from hospital. Hair and fingernail samples continued to show tungsten months later.

Industrial workers exposed to tungsten may develop lung and skin problems. This was the first ever reported case of acute human tungsten poisoning.

The custom of drinking French wine from the just fired barrel of an artillery piece was nothing new. What had happened to the young corporal? An army investigation identified the culprit. Gun barrels recently had been modified to increase the strength of the steel. Tungsten was added. The soldier's comrades had vomited quickly; he had a "steel" stomach. The celebratory practice was halted subsequent to this occurrence.

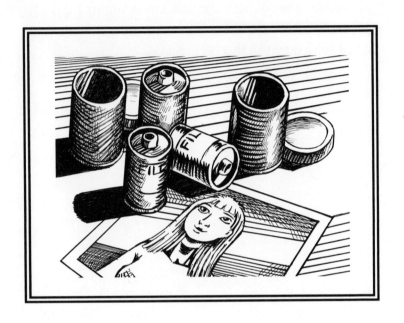

NOT SO SIMPLE APPENDICITIS

A girl of 15 presented to hospital with suspected appendicitis. The appendix is a vestigial remnant of intestine, full of lymphoid tissue. No one is sure what it does. About seven percent of people will develop appendicitis in their lifetime. There is a lower incidence in cultures with high dietary fiber intake, and the condition is more frequent in men than women.

The appendix can become blocked, causing inflammation, and if unchecked it will rupture. It may be blocked by a fecolith, a very small hardened mass of feces mixed with calcium salts, which frequently traverses the bowel. The chance of dying from appendicitis is low, and is more likely to occur in patients who wait too long before presenting to hospital. The same is true of all diseases; the longer you wait, the worse you are likely to do.

. Appendicitis has protean clinical presentations and mimics many other conditions. The classic symptoms are nausea and anorexia, with crampy mid-abdominal pain. The most telling part of the history is migration of the pain from the area around the umbilicus (navel) to the right lower quadrant of the abdomen.

Tamara had a three-day history of abdominal discomfort. She also complained of nausea with vomiting and, according to her mother, had developed a fever. On exam, she was mildly febrile with pain in the right lower quadrant and a positive Rovsing sign (pain in the right lower quadrant when the left lower quadrant is palpated).

A diagnosis of appendicitis was suspected. An appendectomy is a routine operation with a very low complication rate. As a general rule, surgeons operate on these suspected cases knowing some patients will end up having a normal appendix. Operating on the occasional normal patient means the net is cast wide enough to err on the side of caution.

As Tamara's surgery began, there was no reason to expect anything more than a routine procedure. The appendix was easily visualized by the general surgeon. It was normal except at the very tip, which was inflamed. It is odd for only a portion of the appendix to be inflamed; it's usually all or nothing. The tip was adherent to a loop of bowel against which was stuck a fallopian tube and ovary. It was as if a piece of blood-red bubble gum was responsible for this gaggle of organs, sticking them together in an inflammatory mass. As the cut was extended, pus escaped from the knife's incision. An abscess had formed, explaining the young girl's symptoms and physical findings.

As the pus drained, and the area was cleansed with copious amounts of saline, a cylindrical object popped into the surgical field. Where had this come from? It was an empty black 35 mm Kodak film canister with its characteristic gray lid. Its path was tracked on exam, and was found to have migrated through the vaginal wall into the abdomen, where it had formed an abscess and mimicked appendicitis.

The operation was completed. Post-operatively, an intrigued surgeon awaited an explanation from his patient. How had an empty film canister found its way into the belly of his young patient?

An embarrassed teenager recounted how three years previously, she had inserted the film canister into her vagina in an effort to conceal her menstruation. She had been unable to retrieve the plastic cork, and simply forgot about it. It waited three years before deciding to re-appear.

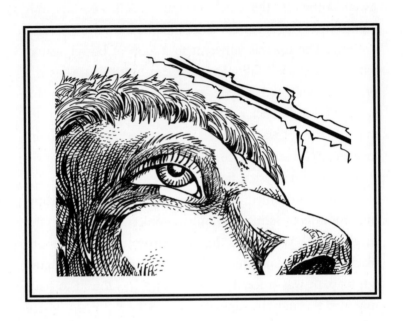

SHOCKING

A 24-year-old man presented to his psychiatrist wishing to stop his anti-depressant medication. He (the patient) had a three-year history of psychotic depression.

During his first year of college, Brian gradually became withdrawn from his surroundings and stopped attending lectures. He shunned contact with his dormitory friends. He was often seen wandering around the university grounds in the middle of the night, unkempt, muttering to himself, and swatting imaginary paper airplanes swirling about his head. After numerous unsuccessful attempts to assist him, his relationship with the university was terminated by the administration.

Brian moved back home with his parents, who lived on a large cattle farm. His condition worsened. He cloistered himself in his room, forbidding his parents to enter. His mother dutifully placed his meals in front of his door, wringing her hands on her apron and praying her only child would recover. He spoke to no one save for unseen ghosts and demons. His appearance became increasingly disheveled. He stopped bathing and brushing his teeth, and his facial expression was constant and dull.

After a month he shunned sunlight, believing he was a vampire. He demanded rare steaks and took to wearing black capes. His bedroom window was covered by black paper. Strange guttural noises emanated from his room at night.

One morning, his father found a cow slaughtered in the yard, blood haphazardly drained from a jagged wound in its neck. The police were contacted and with his tangled oily mess of stringy black hair, Brian was dragged into an ambulance, shouting and spitting. He was carted off to a state psychiatric hospital and remained there, a ward of the state, for months. Diagnosed with psychotic depression, he was filled with medications. Eventually, his condition stabilized with thioridazine pills, weekly intramuscular injections, and maintenance electroconvulsive shock treatments.

After three months, his behavior normalized, and he was discharged in stable condition. He continued to live with his parents, seemingly normal. He landed a job at a fast food restaurant, and felt well, free of hallucinations and delusions.

Brian wanted to stop his medications, but was insightful enough to understand the potential implications to his mental health. He devised and implemented a novel plan. After six months he felt he was ready. He set up an appointment with his psychiatrist to discuss discontinuing his pills.

"Hi," Brian said to the secretary, with a short wave, "I have an 11 o'clock appointment."

"Dr. Houston will be a few minutes," she replied. "Have a seat."

Brian sat in the corner of the waiting room. He was the only patient. Psychiatrists don't like to have more than one patient in the waiting room at a time; it relates to the stigma of mental health. Brian couldn't care less. He was happy and carefree. The waiting room was small, and painted in subtle pinks. The magazine selection was ancient, with back issues of *Time* and *People*.

The secretary noted a pungent aroma of menthol as Brian took a seat.

Dr. Houston came out. He, too, noted menthol in the air. Holding the door knob, he called out to Brian to come into his office, a small and neat room. Books lined a shelf on one wall, a bright picture of a meadow hung on another. Brian sat in the middle of a brown leather couch. Dr. Houston sat in a large deep chair, diagonally placed from his patient. A man of 50, he had short brown hair circling his bald head. His glasses were small, his face long and pointy. He held a pad of lined paper in front of him. Brian's chart rested underneath.

Brian's hair was slicked back. "He looks like Sylvester the Cat," thought Dr. Houston.

He noticed a large red welt in the middle of Brian's forehead. The menthol was pungent in his small office.

"Well Brian, how are you?" he began.

Brian sat there, leaning forward with elbows resting on knees. His smiling face betrayed no hint of awareness of the menthol, which was causing Dr. Houston's eyes to water profusely, or the red welt in the middle of his forehead. It was becoming difficult for Dr. Houston to concentrate on what his patient was telling him.

"I want to stop all of my meds," he said, shouting. "I feel fine, mom and dad aren't worried anymore and they think I'm cured. No more voices or hallucinations Doctor Houston, but I need to know how to stop my meds. Do I taper them or stop them outright?"

"How did you arrive at this?" the doctor asked. "If the

medication is working so effectively, why do you feel a need to discontinue it?"

"I've been experimenting on my own," came the cryptic reply, but he just couldn't help himself. "I might as well tell you. You know how the shock therapy worked so well, and you didn't want to consider maintenance treatments? I decided to do it on my own."

The young man had been administering electroconvulsive shock therapy to himself. Brian had rigged the electrified cattle fence surrounding his parents' farm. He had built a device to control the electric current coursing through the fence. Every week he would crouch in front of the fence, and after bathing his head in menthol, speculating it would improve contact, Brian would touch his forehead to the electric fence. He would invariably fall unconscious, and claimed to feel invigorated and refreshed with each weekly application. His parents supported his assertion of improved mental health, but had no idea how the cattle fence was contributing.

Electroconvulsive therapy (ECT) stimulates the brain with a small electric shock, inducing a brief seizure. This temporarily alters chemical signals in the brain and has been associated with numerous beneficial effects. It has proven to be particularly useful in the treatment of severe depression associated with profound insomnia and suicidal thoughts. It's usually given two or three times per week for 10 sessions. Overnight hospitalization is not necessary for most patients. Recovery is rapid and side effects include brief short-term memory impairment and headaches.

The layperson's view is colored by primitive images of barbaric teeth-clenching shocks administered to patients against their will by Dr. Frankenstein and his assistants. Movies have contributed to caricature representations of this important treatment in psychiatry. There are a number of self-styled "anti-ECT" organizations with the dubious goal of limiting the choice of the mentally ill. ECT has a solid role in the management of severe depression and other forms of mental illness, despite the vociferous pleas of the psychiatrically misinformed with excessive amounts of time on their hands.

Brian's family decided to cut off the electricity to the cattle fence.

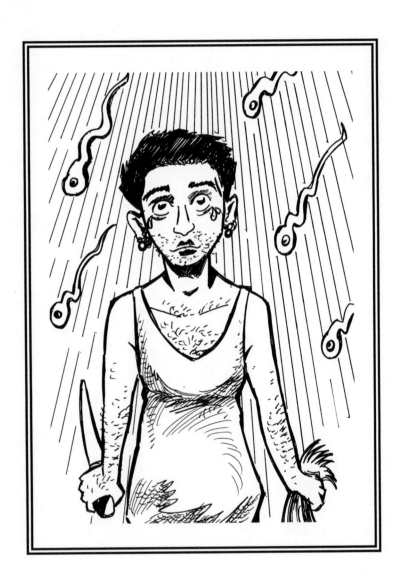

EVERY MAN'S NIGHTMARE

A man arrived in hospital and sat in the triage waiting room.
He needed to talk. Dressed in sky-blue capri pants and a
matching crop top, his breasts heaved rhythmically with
his rapid, shallow breaths. He sat with one leg draped over
the other, ankle swinging anxiously. His nails were filed
square and freshly painted. His hair was too long for his
thin, pointed face. His eyelashes fluttered nervously above
perfectly applied makeup.

The triage room was packed with Saturday night
specials. Drunken and disheveled drug addicts, fat anxious
heart attack patients, and bloodied car accident victims
were wheeled, marched, and dragged into the emergency

department, the severity of their problem jumping them ahead of those less ill. Stephen, or Stephanie as he preferred to be called, wanted to talk. The waiting was killing him, the noise driving him insane. His tortured psyche couldn't deal with the cacophony of the E.R.

After two hours, and a dozen more patients jumping the queue, he brandished the kitchen knife he had brought and ran outside. His mind was in a frenzy. He was angry and confused. His frustration peaked. In the hospital parking lot, he cut himself. He had practiced the strokes a thousand times in his mind, and after waiting five years for surgery, he finally acted upon his impulses.

He yelled out, and like a samurai, fell forward in a pool of rapidly spilling blood. An orderly, Roy, was first on the scene. He was dragging on the last inch of a cigarette, waiting to go back to gurneys and fluid specimens when he witnessed the act of a crazed man/woman, right there in the parking lot.

Roy ran to the E.R. entrance. "Some guy just tried to off himself in the parking lot! He's bleeding bad."

The triage nurse, like a shark sensing drops of blood in the water, grabbed a gurney and enlisted Roy's help, pushing it through a path of startled patients. What she found did not shock her. There was Stephanie, lying on his side in a fetal position, low guttural groans emanating from his throat. He was surrounded by a pool of bright red blood pumping from his groin.

Off to the side, like two misshapen golf balls, lay his testicles. Stephen was a transsexual, and tired of waiting for the government to move forward with his surgery to become an anatomical Stephanie, he decided to take matters into his own hands in an act of self-castration. On closer inspection, his member was lacerated, but he had been too shocked by the sudden extravasation of blood to finish the job.

As a child Stephen was plagued by gender identity issues. As he entered his teenage years, he was convinced he was a woman trapped in a man's body. Stephen had started taking estrogen eight years previously. Breast augmentation surgery had helped assuage his intense need to become a woman, but he felt cursed by his manhood. He would never be a woman until he had rid himself of Bob and the boys.

Thankfully, the testicular artery is an end artery. It meanders no further than the testicles. When transected, the artery will close off in a spasm of constriction. Life-threatening hemorrhage is unlikely. Stephen was treated and released from hospital. He avoided all medical follow-up. Most acts of self-mutilation occur during a psychotic state. Whether Bob followed the fate of the boys is unknown.

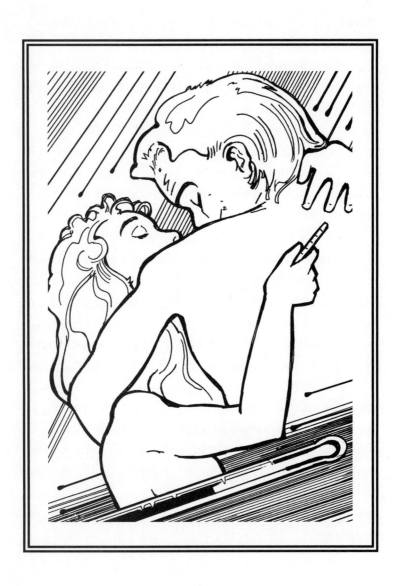

A MISPLACED
THERMOMETER

A nulliparous woman (never having borne a child) of 36 wanted a baby. After over a decade pursuing her career, she was shocked to discover children at the top of her checklist. After a month-long search, she found a husband and embarked on a pregnancy quest. Four months of unsuccessful and often mechanical attempts at impregnation passed. She began measuring her temperature in the early morning, soon after arising, in hopes of improving her odds of conceiving.

Ovulation refers to the release of an egg from a woman's ovaries. The egg is released from one of two ovaries, in response to the body's hormonal signals. It travels down a fallopian tube anticipating a stream of eager sperm to compete for its outer shell. Unlike sperm, tens of millions of which are produced in the testes every month, a woman is born with a finite number of eggs. She cannot increase her allotted number, but there are more than enough to last until her fertility dissipates at menopause.

Ovulation is associated with a slight rise in body temperature. An ancient and thus inexact method for a woman to determine optimum "ripeness" is daily temperature charting. Temperature can be measured from many different places. When it rose, the clothes came off. Her husband, however, was tiring of perfunctory morning sex with his wealthy bride.

In the middle of June, too early on a Saturday to play with thermometers, the alarm clock wailed. Groggy and disheveled, she took the thermometer from the top drawer of her night table. Her husband sleepily hoped she was hypothermic.

She sat at the edge of her bed and went through her ritual. She read in *Cosmopolitan* the previous month that vaginal recordings were the most accurate reflection of core body temperature. Even subtle rises, perhaps one- or two-tenths above normal, could reflect an opportunity to expand her womb, according to the "expert." With half-closed eyelids, she inserted the probe. She waited a minute, heard the beep beep of its circuitry, and went to remove it and check the reading. Her eyes shot open in surprise. She let out a short, quiet gasp.

"The thermometer," she said. "The thermometer," she repeated feverishly. "Edwin, I can't find the thermometer."

Edwin lazily raised his head a few inches off his saliva stained pillow. "Good," he thought.

"Edwin, I put the thermometer in and I can't find it," she whined.

"Well, I'm not searching for it, I might impale myself," he said.

She rushed to the bathroom, and using a special mirror she had purchased years before at a feminist symposium, looked about. No thermometer.

"Maybe it dropped out," she thought. Now fully alert, she raced back to her bedside and with her face only inches above the plush beige carpet, she worked her hands across the floor. No thermometer.

"Get dressed, Edwin!" she yelled. "The thermometer is stuck inside me, we have to get to the doctor."

"Why do *we* have to go," he pleaded. "It's Saturday, I want to sleep. You go and I'll meet you there later."

"Get up, Edwin," she said in a short, low voice, through

clenched teeth. Edwin got up, reluctantly and obediently.

She went to a walk-in clinic and braved the chuckles of the secretary as she relayed her story. In the exam room, she jumped onto the table and placed her feet in the stirrups. The doctor took out the steel speculum and went looking. Nothing.

"I can't find anything," he said. "Are you sure you lost it?"

"I'm positive," she said impatiently. "It must be in there, there's nowhere else it can be. I checked the carpet, I checked the bathroom. It must be there. I can feel it."

"I'll send you for an x-ray downstairs," said the doctor lightheartedly. "At least we can confirm it isn't somewhere in your bedsheets."

An x-ray confirmed the mercury thermometer's position, lying transversely in the pelvis. But where was it? The doctor examined her once again, and neither digital nor speculum examination of her vagina could locate the slippery tool. Finally he decided to arrange a pelvic ultrasound.

There was the thermometer, neatly located in her urinary bladder. In the fogginess of morning, she had inserted it in the wrong place.

A urologist was consulted. A general anesthetic was administered to the patient and the thermometer was removed with an instrument called a cystoscope. The lady was advised to either measure her temperature orally, or ensure she was adequately alert if she wished to maintain intra-vaginal measurements.

Nine months later she gave birth to twins.

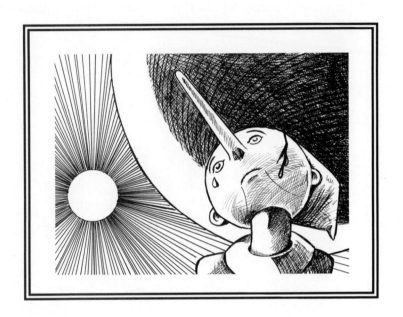

BLOODLESS
TRAUMA

A 27-year-old man was working on a construction job in the early hours of a Sunday morning. It was 4 a.m. and the crew were tiring from hours of labor on the highway. Some were drunk, others stoned, and many both. Breaks were becoming more frequent, but Reggie kept working. Neither drunk nor stoned, Reggie enjoyed the early morning quiet.

As the rest of the crew sat by the side of the road, half-asleep, they heard Reggie cry out. Staggering over to him and barely aware of the occasional passing car, they found him lying face down at the side of the road.

"A car hit him," slurred one of the men. "Call an ambulance, he's not moving. Reggie, Reggie!"

But there was no response. "He's dead," said one of the group of eight workers, swigging from his beer bottle.

"Where the hell's the car?" asked another, rushing to the side of his fallen buddy. "The bastard didn't stop."

Reggie remained face down, unconscious or dead.

One of them went to turn him over. "Don't move him, you idiot," came a shout. "I saw it on TV. You could kill him."

"He's probably dead anyway, and we're gonna catch shit for drinking. Get rid of the damn bottles."

The ambulance arrived moments later. Two caffeinated paramedics jumped out of their vehicle and moved towards the lifeless figure. He was breathing, had a pulse, and his blood pressure was normal.

"I don't see any signs of trauma," said one of them.

"Must be a blunt injury, or more likely his brain is mush. Let's roll out of here," replied his partner as he stepped on fresh shards of broken glass.

They hooked him up to two large intravenous lines, and he winced as the needles found their mark. It was his first sign of life since he had cried out at the impact. Police were on the scene and cordoned off the area. The cops hoped traces of car paint would give away the make and model. Hit and run on a Sunday morning. Probably a drunk driver weaving home from a party.

The crew were interviewed and sent home. The stories

were varied. It was a green BMW, or a black Corvette. One said he saw a transport truck barrel into him, but there was no blood. The cops recognized the intoxication of the crew.

The emergency room was quiet. The trauma phone rang and the team was updated: "Male, about 25, hit working on the highway. Unconscious, no verbal response, no motor response. Two IVs, no airway, ETA 10 minutes."

Upon arrival the information was confirmed. His Glasgow coma scale was five out of 15. The Glasgow coma scale was devised in . . . Glasgow. It is a measure of neurologic injury, and most often utilized in trauma patients. It's a three-category system measuring motor response to commands, speech, and stimuli. The lower the number, the worse the prognosis for neurologic recovery.

Reggie had no speech, no movement, nothing. He reeked of alcohol. There he lay in the trauma room, a dozen health care workers fluttering around him, yet there was no apparent injury. As part of the routine assessment, x-rays were taken of his spine, chest, and pelvis. All were unremarkable. The doctor on duty felt it must have been a severe head injury, but couldn't explain the absence of external trauma. He sent him for a CAT scan of his head. He had seen numerous drivers come in as traumas, who suffered a sudden heart attack or stroke before driving their cars into the nearest tree or ditch.

Maybe Reggie had a seizure or something, but the CAT scan was normal.

After 30 minutes, he seemed to improve. He was mumbling with minimal coherence, "the car . . . the car . . . look out . . . the lights."

Something wasn't right. An experienced nurse, who may very well have seen it all, lifted the seemingly paralyzed arm above Reggie's face, and dropped it. With true paralysis, this is a mild form of torture, for you cannot prevent the arm from smacking into your face.

Reggie's arm miraculously altered its path just before it was to land on his nose. An involuntary protective reflex. She repeated her maneuver, as everyone looked on, with the same result. Most simply left the room to tend to the truly ill.

His spinal collar was removed and he was confronted. "OK Reggie, get up and stop wasting our time. Obviously you're faking it."

Reggie was now awake and alert but protested that he had no recollection of the night, except for a car and headlights bearing down on him. His audience was gone, aside from a pair of interested policemen considering charging him. Reggie left the hospital accompanied by his girlfriend, limping down the hallway.

A review of clinical records from four surrounding

hospitals was telling. He had 23 admissions over eight years for diseases that were never confirmed. Two months earlier, he had been caught mixing blood into his urine, thereby affording an immediate discharge after reappraisal of his entrance complaint of bloody urine. Only five months before, he was admitted to another hospital claiming he had been run over twice by a truck. Reggie had Munchausen syndrome.

Munchausen syndrome was first described in 1951. Baron Von Munchausen was a 19th-century traveler who boasted of fanciful journeys with elaborate stories. Patients who claim to have medical conditions without evidence of organic pathology are likely to have this form of psychiatric pathology.

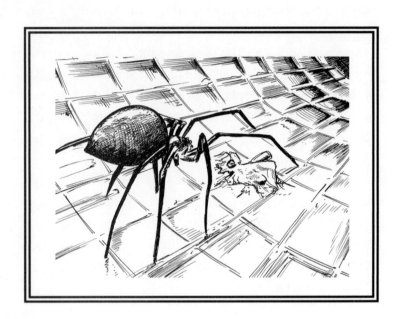

HAPPILY EVER
AFTER

A wealthy 75-year-old man presented to hospital with a variety of neurologic complaints. He had been sick for three months and was getting worse. He had fever, spots on his chest x-ray, abdominal pain, diarrhea, profound weakness, and a peripheral sensory neuropathy, meaning he had trouble feeling his arms and legs.

There was a flurry of diagnostic possibilities handed down from the specialists. Nothing fit as well as hoped. He was pumped with antibiotics and steroids, infused with vitamins and medicine. After a month in hospital, he had improved and was discharged home to the loving care of his wife, Anna.

A month passed and he returned to hospital. His symptoms were back with increasing and alarming severity. He could barely walk, as his proprioceptive sense was gone. Proprioception allows you to know where each body part is in space, with eyes closed. It is known as position sense. It's difficult to walk if you can't "feel" your legs in space. He was wheeled into hospital by his young wife, who then left him to care for their small children.

His reflexes were absent and he couldn't feel his hands and feet. He was gaunt and hollow, his speech a hoarse whisper. He was in pain, but mentally alert. He bent over with abdominal discomfort and continued to have frequent bouts of watery diarrhea.

Lab tests showed pancytopenia, meaning all elements of his blood count were low: red cells (anemia), white cells, and platelets. His blood film showed anisopoikilocytosis, basophilic stippling, irregular pyknotic nuclei, and Howell-Jolly bodies (all not good!). The most unusual physical exam findings were transverse white lines across the nails of his fingers and toes (called Mee's lines), and hard thick skin on his palms and soles (termed hyperkeratosis).

With further interviewing, he reluctantly expressed his belief that his wife was trying to kill him. He had married a woman nearly 50 years his junior, and she quickly bore him three children. Their care was supervised by an army of nannies and other caregivers. She was constantly away, and slept in a separate bedroom. Her nights were long, and never spent in the company of her family. A year previously he arranged for a private investigator to follow her, and, not surprisingly, mountains of evidence of infidelity with many men (and women) were produced. When confronted, she threatened to separate him from his children, asserting that no court would place custody in the hands of one so old and feeble.

He desperately tried to hang onto his young family, and when she started to cook his meals, he felt as if he was making headway. Then the sickness started. At first disbelieving, he reconciled himself to the obvious. She was responsible.

A battery of tests followed, including chemical analysis of his hair, urine, and nails. The diagnosis: arsenic poisoning. After intensive questioning by the local constabulary, Anna admitted the obvious. She had added liberal amounts of arsenic to his evening meals for months. Where she obtained the arsenic was never determined; however it was presumed to originate from insecticides.

The patient underwent chelation treatment. Chelation involves the intravenous administration of a compound called EDTA, which binds heavy metals including arsenic. The EDTA-arsenic combination is then excreted in the urine. Chelation is touted as an alternative treatment for certain forms of heart disease, but is very expensive and has never been proven beneficial.

The Canadian court system decided the children's best interest would be served by awarding full custody to the mother, with no visitation rights and $360,000 a month in alimony and support. The source of the man's toxic levels of arsenic was never explained, and his wife was never charged.

Arsenic is found naturally in the earth's crust. It can be either inorganic or organic, depending on what substances it's combined with. Inorganic arsenic is used as a wood preservative, and organic arsenic is used in insecticides. In some countries, it is used in livestock feed to "fatten" animals. Some scientists believe it is essential for normal human function, in very small amounts. In Victorian England, it was commonly used as a medicinal, packaged as "Dr. Fowler's solution." Because it's naturally present in the ocean, sea animals, especially prawns and oysters, have higher amounts.

Arsenic levels can be measured in blood, nails, and hair, where it accumulates. It may also deposit in organs, and has been linked to tumors in children, especially of the kidney. Toxicity from chronic arsenic ingestion leads to very non-specific symptoms, making a diagnosis extremely difficult.

The old man stopped working and gave his fortune to charity.

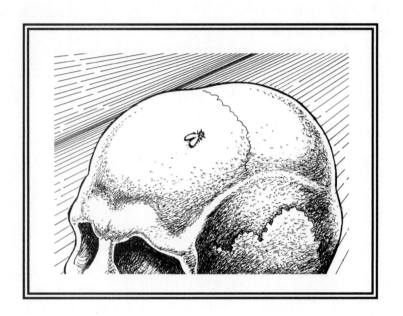

SEVERE INSECT BITES

*A 42-year-old woman returned early from a planned four-*month stay in her native Jamaica after developing fever, chills, malaise, and painful sores on her scalp. While in Jamaica, she suffered from numerous insect bites on her head. The sores healed poorly and became painful and itchy. After a few weeks, small ulcers developed. She felt a rustling sensation each time she tried to sleep. She visited a doctor in Kingston and was prescribed antibiotic ointment and pills. The medication didn't work, her suffering continued, and she decided to cut short her stay and seek medical attention at home.

After an uncomfortable flight, she took a taxi to the

university hospital. In the emergency room she was obviously unwell with tachycardia (fast heart rate), mild hypotension (low blood pressure), and rapid breathing. Her temperature was elevated. She was admitted to hospital with suspected septicemia (bacterial blood infection) and was started on intravenous penicillin and gentamycin. Her infected scalp was the likely source.

After three days, her scalp remained red with three large, black, and necrotic ulcers at the top. It was intensely painful to touch, and her screams filled the hospital ward each time a finger touched her scalp.

"Don't touch my head!" she shrieked. "It's bloody painful. The rustling is drivin' me crazy. I feel like there's somethin' movin' in there."

"Sorry love," replied the nurse. "It's all in your head. I've got to clean it."

The nurse tried to subdue her nausea as she cleansed and bandaged the soft black lesions on the patient's scalp. Despite days of antibiotics and wound care, the fever continued. A decision was made to take her to the operating room for surgical debridement (removal of dead and decaying tissue) of her infected scalp.

In the operating room the following day, a general surgeon draped her scalp and cleansed the area with betadine. He incised the ulcerated areas and began the debridement. As he reached in with a steel curette to scrape out dead tissue, his eyes caught a flash of movement. To his horror and disgust, the curette exited the wound with a wriggling fly larvae impaled on its end.

He had discovered a larval infestation deep within her scalp. She was full of bugs. A surgical scrub nurse rushed out of the operating theater to toss her cookies. A basin was brought forward and hesitantly handed to the surgeon. He thought about dropping them on the floor and squishing them with his surgical clogs. Instead, he conquered his initial queasiness and casually plucked larvae after larvae from deep within her head. After an exhausting two hours, the tally was 44. The larvae were forwarded to the entomology department of the university and identified as *Cochliomyia hominivorax*, also known as the New World screwworm, a type of fly. She recovered from the sepsis; however the destruction of her scalp was severe enough to require reconstructive plastic surgery. The likely sequence was a minor infection of her scalp, followed by colonization by the fly larvae and further infection extending beyond the scalp.

Human infestation by fly larvae is called *myiasis*. Larvae either require a living host (obligate) or may develop in a dead host (facultative). Some insects, such as the bot fly, can penetrate intact skin. The egg-laying females of others may infest pre-existing wounds, as in this case.

The woman required psychiatric assessment after developing a fear of insects.

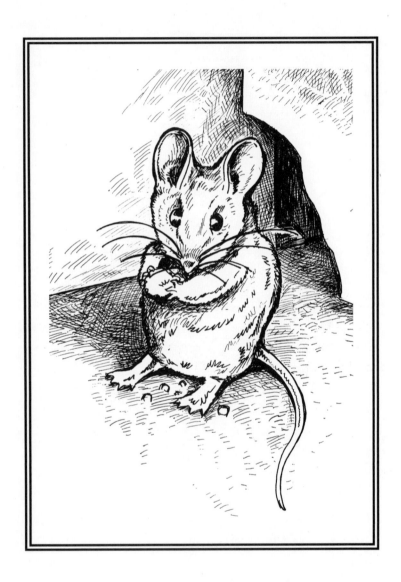

A RUNNY NOSE

Charlene was at the end of her shift, tending to the sick and dying in the intensive care unit (ICU). In an ICU, one nurse is assigned to one patient. Charlene's unfortunate patient on this shift was a 79-year-old woman who had suffered a heart attack at home. When the ambulance had arrived, her heart had stopped. No one at the scene was able to perform CPR, leaving her with inadequate cerebral blood flow for five minutes.

Although she recovered some neurologic function, improvement was minimal, and four weeks later she remained on a breathing machine, a few steps ahead of a vegetable. The doctors were having difficulty convincing the distraught family that ongoing medical care was futile, and were preparing to "pull the plug" the following day, against the wishes of the next-of-kin.

"This is ridiculous," Charlene thought. "I feel like I'm looking after a dead patient. What's the point?" She swatted at the flies. For a month the nurses had been complaining of flies buzzing around the unit.

Charlene was at the foot of the bed in a black swivel chair busily writing in the chart, when her peripheral vision noted movement. She looked up at her patient. At first she thought the discharge moving from her patient's nose and down her face was simply a runny booger. As she moved closer to clean it, she shrieked and ran out of the room.

Shaking and frightened, she directed her colleagues to the bedside.

"What the hell is coming out of her nose?" she wailed.

Crawling in an orderly single file was a line of squirming maggots. White, plump, and juicy, they disappeared into her mouth. A few other nurses screamed, one lost consciousness, and the ICU was in an uproar.

"There's bugs in her nose!" a nurse screamed. "She's infested with maggots." Phone calls were already placed to the union's insurance company for mental disability forms.

A brave doctor was summoned (ordered) to check out the bizarre infestation. Attaching a catheter to wall suction, he confidently strode to the patient's side, shoved the catheter up her nose, and turned on the suction. As a half-dozen maggots flew out of her nose and mouth into the collection bag, he vomited.

Public relations was desperately trying to contain the event. Later that day, an ear nose and throat surgeon was called. Dressed in a white lab coat, he inserted a scope into her nose, the abode of the maggots. He glimpsed and grasped the one remaining insect larvae, inspected the rest of the nasopharyngeal cavity, and declared it fumigated, free of infestation.

He had barely packed up his equipment, when a scream emanated from the next room. A nurse fled from another patient's room. More maggots. The entire ICU was closed down, and each patient was inspected for maggot infestation. No other cases were identified.

The maggots were sent to the entomology department, and identified as the green blowfly. The entomologist was intrigued and decided to sleuth out the problem. Under the assumption that a few electric fly traps would suffice, the hospital administration spurned his offer of assistance.

Despite the traps, the staff continued to notice flies in the ICU and hospital corridors. When local newspapers discovered the embarrassing problem, the entomologist was called. As he toured the hospital and basement, he noted a large number of mouse carcasses. He had found the source.

A month previously, the hospital was plagued by mice. The infestation was thought to be related to a reduction in housekeeping staff. Mice were often seen scampering through the hospital wards, and in a few instances were being cared for as pets by staff. Glue boards and traps laced with warfarin were set. Because of the staff shortage, the traps were not cleared of the dead mice. The mice carcasses attracted blowflies, which, in addition to laying eggs in the mice, subjected the ICU patients to the blowflies' breeding habits. A thorough search of the hospital was undertaken, and carcasses were removed. Live traps were set, and nearly 200 mice were captured. The mouse/blowfly problem seemed to have been solved until a year later, when blowflies were found in surgical wounds. A search of the operating rooms uncovered further dead mice that had been missed a year earlier.

A mouse carcass is a potential home for up to 100 blowfly eggs. When the blowflies entered the ICU, attracted to the hospital because of the ready availability of mouse meat, there was no way out because of the automatic doors protecting the ICU. Without the mice, the flies laid eggs in the next best place, the nasal discharge of ill patients.

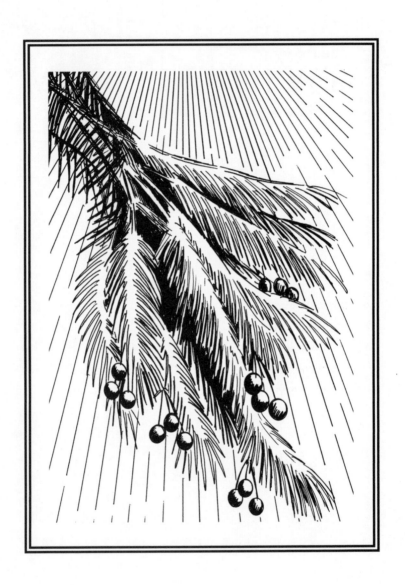

YEW NEVER KNOW

A young man of 18 was taken to hospital via ambulance. He was found in a park unconscious. His blood pressure was dangerously low and a central line was inserted into his right external jugular vein. After two quick liters of normal saline, his blood pressure normalized.

An intravenous comes in a sterile package, and is made up of a hollow steel needle within a plastic catheter with a blunt end. The steel needle is longer than the plastic catheter. This allows the venipuncturist to poke the vein with the needle first, and then slide the catheter over it, so that all that remains in the vein is a soft and flexible plastic catheter. Intravenous lines have different internal calibers, termed the gauge. An 18" gauge needle is wider than a 21" gauge one and allows fluid to infuse at a much faster rate.

Above a certain gauge, the limitation to flow rate is the size of the vein — particularly relevant when a patient arrives in hospital with dangerously low blood pressure. Since trauma patients may extravasate liters of blood from wounds and crushed organs, rapid infusion of blood, saline, and albumin is crucial. But an arm vein does not allow enough fluid to infuse.

The solution is a central line. Examples of large veins are the external jugular vein, subclavian vein (below the collarbone), and femoral vein (in the leg). The 18-year-old was stuck in the neck with a big needle.

He improved neurologically, but could not follow verbal commands. His heart rate fluctuated wildly from 30 to 250 beats per minute. En route to the intensive care unit, his monitor showed erratic and disorganized electrical activity. He was defibrillated with 300 joules of electricity, with no effect. A tube was inserted into his lungs and he was hooked up to a ventilator.

Despite repeated electrical shocks, his heart did not respond. A temporary pacemaker, used to activate his heart muscle, was inserted through the right femoral vein. Again his heart did not respond. Cardiopulmonary resuscitation continued and over the next two hours he was shocked, paced, ventilated, and infused with every emergency medication stocked in the hospital's pharmacy. There was marginal improvement. An intentional overdose was suspected.

A nurse was foraging through the man's pockets, a common procedure to identify a comatose patient and perhaps find a cocaine rock or ecstasy tablet. She came across pine needles and small red berries. She recognized them as originating from the yew tree (*Taxus baccata*).

The following day he exhibited dramatic improvement. Awake, alert, and sitting in bed, his only complaint was a sore chest from the CPR. After denying attempted suicide, he admitted to frequently ingesting plants, with his secure knowledge that all things natural were healthy. He was cautioned to avoid this practice. Within 18 hours of admission, and near death many times, he was discharged after being cleared by the psychiatry service.

Yew is a well-known toxin in veterinary medicine. Animals often ingest yew needles and berries. In a German zoo there was a spate of emu deaths. The zookeepers noticed the birds were poking their beaks through the fencing to eat the yew trees growing on the outside.

In the 19th century, yew was considered a medicinal to eradicate worms. There were many reports of intoxication. Recently, four Polish prisoners drank a mixture of boiled yew needles, and three died, exhibiting the same cardiac toxicity shown by this patient. Yew contains diterpinoid alkaloids, responsible for the extreme cardiac toxicity of this plant.

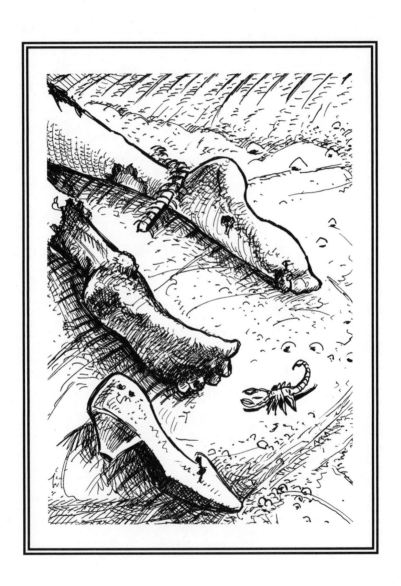

AUTOEROTIC
DEATH

A 36-year-old man was found dead in the middle of the Australian Outback in 106 degree Fahrenheit (41C) temperature.

Two hikers had found a small river near the trail they were navigating. Sweaty and spent, their attention turned to a refreshing swim in the potentially crocodile laden waters. Divesting themselves of boots, socks, and clothes, they jumped into the warm waters, and within minutes were in the midst of a passionate interlude. Fumbling to the rocky shore, their desire culminating in satisfaction, James let out a startled cry.

"Sean, look!" he shrieked, pointing to the motionless

and dessicated corpse lying on an outcrop of large boulders 10 feet away. A pair of blood-red pumps had tumbled from the body's shrivelled feet onto the desert floor. The frightened couple collected themselves, and quickly dressed. They cautiously approached the mummified remains, clinging to each other for safety.

"Ewww, it's gross, he's dead. He looks like he's been here for decades. What are we going to do?" asked James.

"I don't know. Just calm down. Don't panic," replied Sean. "Get your cell phone out of your pants. We can call the police," he suggested.

The area was cordoned off 40 minutes later when the police force from the local town arrived at the scene in two clouds of dust. A policeman slowly exited his car, and, dragging his hefty frame through the desert heat, bent over the body.

"It's gotta be Hank," said the constable, smoking a cigar. "He's been missing for almost a year."

It was definitely Hank. Hank was a high school science teacher in a tiny farming community of 500 in the Australian Outback. Despite an intensive month-long search after his sudden disappearance a year before, the issue was unsolved until the hikers chanced upon his remains.

He was dressed in expensive women's lingerie, and half a dozen pairs of pantyhose. The underwear was cut to expose his genitals. It appeared Hank may not have been the best role model for the town's impressionable youth. It was presumably difficult for Hank to indulge in his fantasy life within the town, but relatively simple on the outskirts. Death was likely the result of heat-stroke.

Autoerotic death is defined as accidental death during attempts at sexual satisfaction. Ropes or scarves used as ligatures during sexual escapades may be an unfortunate cause of asphyxiation. Many a hapless corpse has been diagnosed with autoerotic death. Autoerotic deaths may occur during bizarre sexual practices resulting in compromising and embarrassing post-mortem situations.

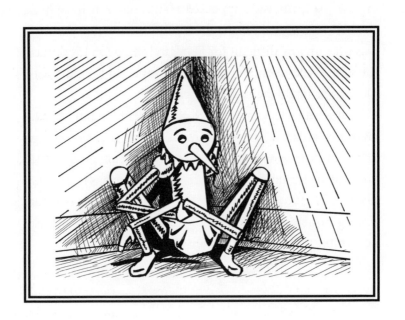

FRACTURES WHERE
THERE IS NO BONE

A 28-year-old man was in the midst of sexual intercourse with his wife when he felt a snap, and heard a crack and a pop. This was followed by severe genital pain. His vigorous thrusts were abruptly truncated and upon examination of his swollen member he observed sudden detumescence. He began to feel lightheaded and nauseous, fearful of what he may have broken.

He fainted, but was easily aroused by his wife. She got him to his feet, bundled him and his member into the car, and drove to the local emergency room.

Next to his name on the triage board was written "fractured penis," for this was exactly the diagnosis. His penis had fractured in the middle, tearing the soft tissue and resulting in a large hematoma around the middle of his flaccid member.

A urologist was called. No blood was evident at the meatus (opening), and despite the urge, the patient was unable to urinate. He was taken to the O.R. and his penis was degloved (skin taken up) and then repaired. Other than mild curvature, there were no other long-term effects from his injury. Erectile function was reported as normal on follow-up.

Penile fractures most often occur during sex. Other mechanisms of injury include excessive masturbatory force and direct blunt trauma. There is even a report of a penile fracture after rolling over in bed. Perhaps the most dreaded complication is a post-operative wound infection resulting in abscess formation, which requires surgical drainage. Erectile dysfunction is uncommon.

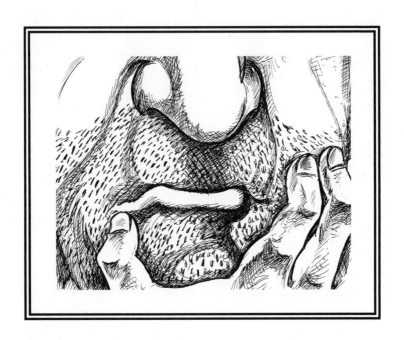

ELECTRIC SHAVINGS

A man of 52 was found dead in his hospital room in the early morning of May 23, 1998. A student nurse arrived for her shift, bouncing cheerily from patient to patient during ward rounds. When she walked into room 36 she discovered the bloated, lifeless body of Carlos Menegez. He lay on his back, the hospital bedsheets half covering his thick hairless legs and enormous shiny belly. Brown lips slightly parted and eyes peering vacantly, he had quietly passed away during the night. His skin was grayish white.

He had been admitted in April with jaundice and liver failure. In end-stage liver failure, the abdomen fills with clear straw-colored fluid, called ascites. Up to 10 liters of fluid may accumulate, resembling pregnancy. Mr. Menegez had severe ascites and leg swelling. A paracentesis was performed, where a needle is inserted into the abdominal cavity and drains fluid. Eight liters were removed the first day, and, as expected, reaccumulated rapidly. Liters more were removed twice a week.

For a decade he had suffered from a movement disorder marked by a constant tremor of his hands, diagnosed as Parkinson's disease. He gave a history of mildly excessive alcohol use. The doctors guessed this was the cause of his liver failure.

Investigations included an abdominal ultrasound and blood tests of his liver function. There was no evidence of exposure to any of the various hepatitis viruses, and his liver had evolved into a shrunken fibrotic scar. He was diagnosed with hepatic cirrhosis (cirrhosis of the liver).

Weeks after admission, his hospital course was complicated by pneumonia. His family was attentive and supportive as his condition deteriorated. As his kidneys failed, the family elected to assign him DNR status (Do Not Resuscitate) so that no heroic measures would be performed to prolong his agony. Days later he was found dead. His death certificate listed pneumonia, alcoholic cirrhosis, and Parkinson's as the cause of death. At the family's request, no autopsy was performed and he was cremated. His ashes were scattered on the soccer pitch he had loved as a youth.

Years later, his 35-year-old son, now a successful doctor, asked to re-examine his father's death. The file was reopened and at the son's suggestion a genetic condition called Wilson's disease was entertained as a possible cause of death.

Wilson's disease (hepatolenticular degeneration) is a genetic disorder that prevents the body from removing copper. A protein in the blood called ceruloplasmin removes copper. In Wilson's disease, ceruloplasmin levels are reduced and copper accumulates in organs causing liver failure and a movement disorder from deposits in the brain. Treatment is chelation (EDTA compound binds the heavy metal and is then excreted) and avoidance of foods containing copper, including chocolate and mushrooms.

Unfortunately, the diagnosis of Wilson's disease is based on genetic testing of tissue. The cremation and subsequent distribution of his ashes made that impossible.

An electric shaver used by Mr. Menegez was found. The last gift his wife had bought him, she was unable to discard it. Small amounts of hair and skin were taken from the shaver, which had been used only by the patient, and were sent for genetic testing. It was confirmed posthumously that he had suffered from Wilson's disease. Had he been diagnosed while alive, treatment may have extended his life.

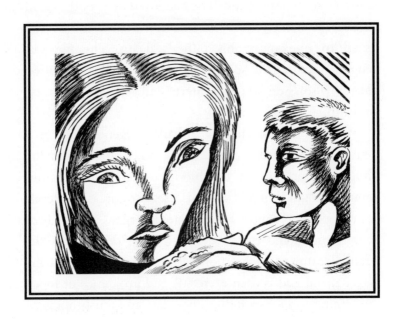

AN ODD ALLERGY

Joni was an attractive woman of 23. She was healthy and active, her only medical history being asthma, which developed at the age of 13. Her condition was mild and easily controlled with bronchodilator and steroid inhalers. Raised in a religious household in a small rural town, she decided at a young age to remain a virgin until her wedding day.

She had met Jay in her senior year of high school. They shared chemistry. Jay was Joni's first love, but she would not consummate until their wedding. They were engaged soon after finishing high school, and married five years later when Jay felt he could support a family.

Jay's calm demeanor hid the frustration of a young man denied. He told Joni he respected her stance on pre-marital sex, but it took every manly bone in his body not to coerce her into a roll in the hay. After many long and difficult years, the wedding arrived. Jay had only one thing on his mind, and so did Joni. Despite her strong religious beliefs, she was practically salivating with anticipation of sex with her husband.

The wedding was elaborate, since Joni was an only child. The banquet hall was festooned with pink roses, food and alcohol flowed, and a nine-piece band played until 2 a.m. Jay and Joni wanted to take their leave as early as they could, so that they could consummate their marriage.

At midnight, the limo driver dropped the newlyweds off at their hotel, and they breathlessly rode the elevator to the bridal suite, clawing at each other's clasps, zippers, and buttons.

Within minutes, clothes were piled by the doorway, and the naked couple coupled. It was a short tryst, but they were nonetheless satisfied that the albatross was removed from their necks, and they could begin a life of personal and sexual exploration.

Soon after completion of the "act," Joni began to feel flushed. "Jay, I feel kind of hot," she said.

Jay was not displeased to hear that his new bride

wanted another kick at the can. "Give me a couple of minutes at least hon, we just finished."

"No, I mean I really feel hot, and my skin is getting all blotchy. I'm itchy and it kind of hurts inside."

"What do you mean inside? Inside where?"

"You know, there."

"Go take a bath," came his helpful reply.

A few hours passed and her symptoms abated. Joni was bothered by what had happened to her so soon after her first sexual experience, and decided it must have been from the anticipation of the moment. "Was sex always like this?" she wondered.

The following afternoon, like the newlyweds they were, Jay and Joni were at it again. Soon after completion, Joni developed the same symptoms. This went on for months and was seriously denting their sexual life together. The only available relief was her husband's use of a condom.

After a particularly severe post-coital episode, with ugly red blotches on her limbs and torso, a feeling of throat constriction, and severe vaginal discomfort, she sought help from her doctor. She knew it had something to do with sex but couldn't understand the relationship. Had she upset God in some way? Were her true pre-marital sexual urges somehow responsible for this punishment from the skies? The doctor took a history and performed a physical exam, but found nothing unusual. He referred her to a gynecologist, because of the relationship of her symptoms to sexual intercourse.

The gynecologist had seen it all before and wasted no time in pinpointing the diagnosis. He pronounced her in possession of a hypersensitivity reaction to her husband's seminal fluid. After so many years of patient waiting and anticipation, her one true love harbored an allergenic substance. Joni was allergic to Jay's sperm.

Options included divorce, lifelong condom use, topical intravaginal steroids before intercourse, or topical desensitization. They chose the latter. In topical desensitization, the husband supplies a steady stream of sperm to the lab. Increasing concentrations of sperm are introduced intravaginally every 20 minutes during each session. Jay and Joni were instructed to engage in sex at least three times a week, which was still easy in the early phase of their marriage. After three months, and lots of sex, Joni was able to enjoy normal relations with her husband with no symptoms. Unfortunately, she had yet to figure out an orgasm.

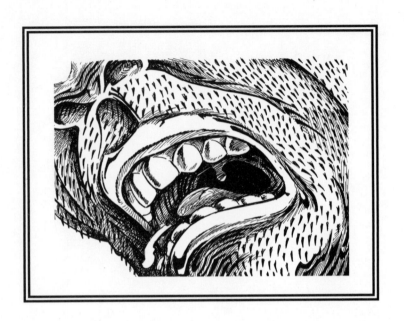

FOREIGN BODY

Scott was a 27-year-old single man. After months of mild, nagging stomach discomfort, he awoke at 3 a.m. with severe, sharp, central abdominal pain. He felt lightheaded and nauseous.

He painfully inched his way across the bed to the phone and dialed 911. "I have horrible pains. . . . Come now," he whispered. He lapsed into unconsciousness before he could respond to the questions fired by the operator.

The ambulance arrived and found Scott lying in bed, barely breathing, and hypotensive (had low blood pressure). He had a tube placed into his throat at the scene to support his breathing. Two large-bore intravenous lines, deftly inserted by the paramedics into his veins, poured saline into his body. His blood pressure picked up and he was whisked to hospital. The ambulance had called the emergency room, allowing precious minutes of preparatory time for the gravely ill man.

"BP 85/50, heart rate 130," the paramedic shouted breathlessly on arrival. "He called 911 and collapsed. When we got there his BP was barely obtainable, but picked up with fluids."

The paramedics delivered their intubated load to the acute room into a waiting circle of doctors, nurses, orderlies, and technicians. They were dressed in matching surgical greens with splash protectors covering their faces. These are used during the management of potentially bloody emergencies.

"His BP is way too low," shouted the emergency team leader. "Crossmatch him for six units and someone call the respiratory tech down, we need this guy hooked up to a vent. I want the surgical fellow down here stat."

Scott was conscious and fighting the discomfort of the breathing tube scratching his pharynx. No sedation was administered for fear of masking the cause of his problem.

Gloved hands probed every inch of him and in him. When they rested on his abdomen, he grimaced and it became involuntarily rigid. He had guarding, a sign of irritation within his abdominal cavity. Something was in there. When his blood count returned with a hemoglobin of 74, he was wheeled out of the emergency room onto the elevator and into the operating theater on the third floor for urgent surgical exploration.

Hemoglobin reflects the number of red blood cells coursing through blood vessels. A fit young man like Scott should have a hemoglobin twice what was recorded. He was bleeding from somewhere in his abdomen. A spontaneous occurrence like this in a 27-year-old man has few causes, all of them rare.

"Perhaps he had a bleeding ulcer," thought the surgeon, as he vigorously scrubbed his arms and hands in preparation for the emergency surgery. With 20 years of experience and countless cases, he had seen it all. His memory recalled a few similar cases in his extensive mental library. A young woman with a ruptured appendix, a boy with an uncontrollable bleed from a duodenal ulcer, and a woman with an ectopic pregnancy all had presented with abdominal pain, hypotension, and anemia.

Blood poured out of Scott's abdomen as the peritoneal cavity was sliced into by the scalpel. Liters cascaded onto the floor like a red waterfall. The surgeon began to perspire. "I can't see anything in here, give me more suction," he barked. The suction catheter sucked the blood rapidly, only to have new pools rapidly coalesce. The surgeon knew this was an even bigger problem than he anticipated.

"Blood pressure's dropping," intoned the anesthetist from the head of the bed, as he controlled the ventilator and monitored vital signs.

"We're pouring blood and platelets into this kid and I can't keep his BP up. I need two units of fresh frozen plasma now," shouted the surgeon. The O.R. was a beehive, with nurses and orderlies scurrying to keep up with the orders like busy waitresses. They were losing him.

The surgeon knew he had only minutes to stop the unseen hemorrhaging. He rapidly explored the abdomen from the inside, shoving aside organs and pinching vessels. Extra suction catheters tried to keep the field clear with marginal success. At last he found it: one of the mesenteric arteries, the blood supply to the intestines, was pouring blood. He nimbly clamped it and the bleeding at once ceased. He had put his finger in the dyke. What he found next surprised him. Poking through either side of the artery was a sharp wooden toothpick. Somehow a toothpick had eroded through Scott's intestines and by an unfortunate turn, had perforated a major intestinal artery.

Later in the ICU, Scott's father recalled driving with his son in Scott's bright red pick-up. He had hit a curve on a country road, and the impact dislodged the toothpick from

Scott's teeth. He had been chewing toothpicks habitually since giving up smoking. Scott wasn't sure where the toothpick fell at the time, and quickly dismissed it. The toothpick had been inadvertently swallowed. Though most foreign bodies find an uneventful passageway through the intestines, if sharp enough some will perforate the lining and cause severe consequences.

Despite the medical team's heroic efforts, Scott had lost too much blood and died two days post-operatively.

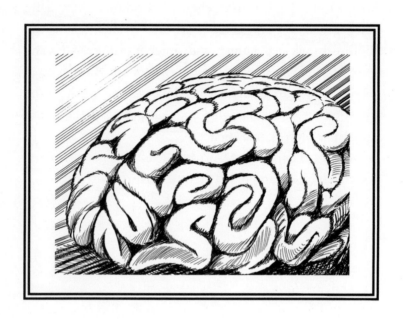

SEXUAL FEELINGS

A 34-year-old woman was referred to a neurologist for investigation of abrupt loss of consciousness (syncope).

While lecturing at a business symposium a week previously, she experienced a sudden and profound feeling beginning deep within her pelvic region and ascending throughout her body. It was indistinguishable from an intense orgasm. This was followed by numbness in her left arm and a rhythmic jerking of her hand. She then collapsed onto the floor and briefly lost consciousness. Her business associates crowded around her as she moaned and writhed on the carpet. An ambulance was summoned. She awoke quickly, and her initial confusion cleared. She refused assistance from the ambulance attendants and, feeling embarrassed, went home.

Over the previous five years, she had almost weekly spontaneous orgasms, albeit without syncope. There was no pattern to their occurrence. All of her orgasms began in the same fashion and without warning. They occurred when grocery shopping, driving in a car, riding an elevator, and eating at restaurants. Her orgasms were characteristically intense and left her strained and anxious. She had learned to stifle outward manifestations of what was transpiring, but had no control over their onset or duration. Though transiently a novelty, she soon loathed these uninvited sensations. She had not told her doctor about them because of her unease.

Her history was otherwise non-contributory. She had no prior hospitalizations and was on no medications. She was married, had three children, and was unable to experience sexual satisfaction during intercourse. Her husband was unaware of either of her dilemmas. The physical examination was entirely unhelpful. Her neurologist thought that the rhythmic jerking of her hand, associated with syncope and orgasms, was due to a sexual seizure disorder.

Brain imaging studies were ordered including computerized axial tomography (CAT scan). A month later she was scheduled for the test, and had an orgasm in the waiting room of the radiology office. The test was completed and a diagnosis was determined.

In the right temporal lobe of her brain, a strange confluence of tangled abnormal blood vessels was identified, termed an arteriovenous malformation (AVM). The temporal lobe of the brain has many functions, including sexual and erotic processing. Her AVM was deep within these brain centers, and its growth triggered increasingly frequent orgasms by stimulating the site that controls this experience. Her diagnosis was sexual seizures due to an AVM of the sexual center of her temporal lobe.

She underwent successful surgery to remove the vascular tumor, and remained orgasm-free. Her husband remained unaware of her dilemma(s).

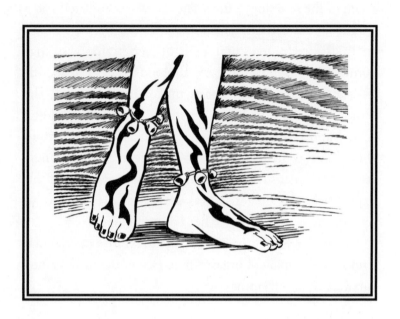

BODY PAINTING

Henna is used throughout the Middle East and Asia as temporary artistic jewelry to enhance beauty. A 36-year-old woman from Saudi Arabia was decoratively applying henna to the soles of her feet when she collapsed into unresponsiveness. She was rushed to the emergency room by numerous distraught relatives.

She was visiting from her native country to attend the wedding of a distant cousin. Neither she nor the wedding party spoke English, thus the history was not entirely clear to the emergency room staff.

Her relatives shouted Arabic in a cacophony of confusion. An interpreter was summoned, but crowd control became difficult, and while doctors worked to diagnose and treat the patient, hospital security was called to control the ever-burgeoning group. A scuffle occurred and a guard was knocked to the ground, prompting two policemen, in the emergency room investigating a car accident, to attempt to defuse the situation. They were shoved and spat upon, and soon dozens of uniformed cops flocked to the scene. Seventeen people were arrested and charged with assault, and deportation was planned. It was going to be a much smaller wedding than anticipated.

One young woman, the patient's daughter, was allowed to remain with her in the acute room to assist the doctors in sorting out the problem. According to the history, obtained through an Arabic interpreter, the mother had spent considerable time applying henna, and after finishing the soles of both feet, began decorating other parts of her body. She soon complained of breathlessness and sought relief by going outside. She got up from her seat, took two or three steps and catapulted forward, striking her face on a table.

In the hospital, it was apparent she was in trouble. Her face bloody and swollen, she was having severe breathing difficulty and was intubated and placed on a mechanical ventilator. Her vital signs were otherwise reasonable, with normal blood pressure and a slightly elevated heart rate.

The henna mixture was a special preparation brought from Saudi Arabia for the event. Two other women had begun using it, and they experienced similar, but less intense breathing symptoms that did not require medical attention.

Her chest x-ray showed white patches throughout both lung fields, consistent with fluid in the lungs (pulmonary edema). There was no indication of a heart attack or any cardiac condition, the most common cause of the x-ray abnormality. She was admitted to the hospital's intensive care unit where she remained for three days before making a complete recovery. No other abnormalities were noted during her stay and the remainder of her investigations proved normal.

As no other cause could be identified, and the incident was temporarily related to the henna application, her doctors pursued their only lead.

Henna is a dye. Another dye, known as para-phenylene-diamine (PPD), is added to hasten the process of dyeing and to improve the definition of the intricate designs. The substance is highly toxic when absorbed into the body, and has been associated with numerous suicides. It causes respiratory problems, and many other severe reactions including renal failure and muscle breakdown. The dye is banned in most countries. Undoubtedly, after using so much henna, the PPD was absorbed into the woman's body resulting in the clinical picture of respiratory distress. The Saudi Arabian source of the PPD was identified and the remainder of the stash confiscated. Whether or not the "supplier" was beheaded is unknown.

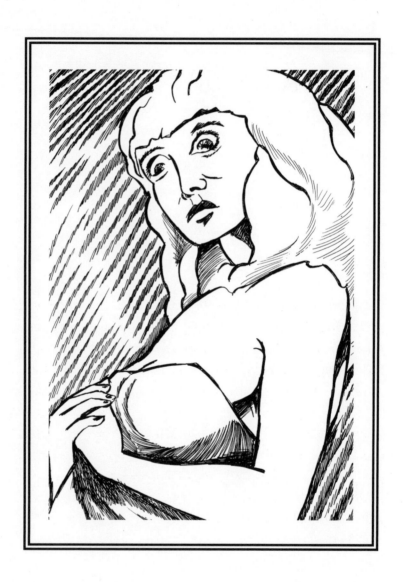

A STRANGE PLEURAL EFFUSION

Marge was an attractive and shapely woman of 54. Thrice divorced, with four grown children, she enjoyed partying like a teenager. Aware she was openly flirtatious, her friends always kept one eye on their husbands when Marge was around. She wore form-fitting blouses, tight jeans, and hoop earrings. Her fingers were clad in diamonds and gold. A cigarette always dangled from her heavily painted lips. Wisps of smoke wound through her curly orange hair.

"Something's wrong," she told her boyfriend after a particularly vigorous love-making session. "At the end there, I was getting some chest pressure."

"Is it still there?" he drawled, puffing on his cigarette.

"It's easing up a bit," she replied. The discomfort gradually ebbed and after another five minutes, was gone.

Over the next few weeks, the chest pressure recurred. It began as an exertional symptom, and was soon awakening her from sleep. Her 35 years of cigarette use had caught up with her; she was suffering from angina. After appointments and tests, she was diagnosed with severe coronary artery disease. The blood vessels of her heart were narrowed and damaged, and bypass surgery was required. Marge's greatest fear was the cosmetic effects of a scar on her buxom chest. She resigned herself to the operation, and quit smoking soon after the diagnosis.

The surgery went well. Her sternum was wired shut and the skin was closed with staples. Bilateral chest tubes were inserted, a routine feature of all bypass surgeries. Chest tubes are flexible plastic conduits placed in the space around each lung, called the pleural space. The tubes are often inserted below the ribs at the front of the chest, just below the breasts.

Coronary bypass is a major surgical procedure. In otherwise healthy patients, the mortality rate is three percent. Convalescence requires months. The first week is the hardest, and patients are rarely strong enough to return home earlier.

Marge's recovery was characteristically difficult. Her

first few days spent in the cardiovascular intensive care unit were a nightmarish haze of discomfort. Her chest ached, it was painful to take deep breaths, and tubes seemed to draw fluid from every orifice of her body. Despite her aches, she gradually rose from her bed. Marge graduated from small steps to walks around the ward. Her shortness of breath seemed to persist. Her doctors attributed it to the normal effects of major cardiac surgery.

After one week she returned home. Her chest healed, but she still found herself straining to breathe with minimal activities. She had lost 20 pounds, and her curvaceous figure had flattened out. Her right breast in particular seemed to have lost its poise. Though Marge was confused, the pain of recovery did not allow her to focus on her vanity, as she struggled with her daily activities.

After four weeks, Marge was seen by her cardiovascular surgeon in follow-up. A chest x-ray confirmed a persistent and large right pleural effusion. It is very common for fluid to accumulate around one or both lungs after heart surgery. This is an inflammatory process, in response to the irritation of the operation.

The fluid would have to come out and the surgeon made arrangements for a brief hospital stay. Marge leaned forward in her hospital bed. Her back was prepped with sterile solution, and draped with surgical green towels. A small needle injected anesthetic. A second needle, only slightly larger than the first, was inserted between her ribs into the pleural space. As the surgeon pulled back on the syringe, he met resistance. No matter how many times he tried, the same problem occurred. Pleural fluid is usually the consistency of water or blood. It should easily pass through a needle unless loculated.

Using a larger needle, he tried again, with greater success. The liquid that filled the syringe surprised him; it was yellow, pasty, and viscous, like molasses. He was unable to remove more than a few milliliters, though he was certain from the x-ray that far more was there.

The material was sent to the pathology lab and reviewed under the microscope. The result: crystals of silicone. Marge's silicone breast implant had ruptured into the space around her lungs. This probably occurred when the chest tubes were first inserted immediately after surgery. Her right silicone implant was likely nicked, and silicone tracked into the pleural space through the large tube.

Marge was admitted, a second chest tube was required to drain her breast from her chest, and she was sent home lopsided. Two months later, she underwent yet another operation, this time by a plastic surgeon to balance her assets.

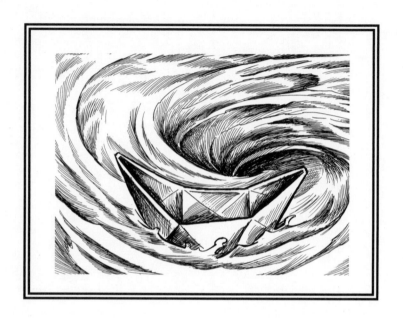

SUCTION

Arnie was a rambunctious 15-year-old boy who loved playing sports. It was summertime, and with the advent of global warming, an August heat wave was in full force when he called up Benny, his best friend.

"Let's go to the pool for a swim," said Arnie, dripping sweat onto the linoleum floor of the kitchen. The AC was down, and he couldn't stay indoors any longer. It was only 9 a.m.

"Sounds good," replied Benny, Froot Loops spilling out of his mouth. "I just gotta finish breakfast. You want to meet me there, or should I pop by?"

"I'll meet you there in 30 minutes," said Arnie, and he hung up the phone.

Arnie grabbed a Gatorade and pedaled his bike to the public swimming pool. It was loaded with early morning arrivals, parents and their kids staking their claims on the narrow concrete surrounding the pool. Bright towels dotted the grounds.

Arnie secured an open spot near the deep end, laid down his towel in a territorial gesture, and dove in the frigid water. He had been swimming since he was five, and comfortably lapped the pool a few times. He submarined to the bottom, and tried swimming the length of the pool underwater. Arnie touched the tiles on the side of the shallow end and his head broke the surface. He breathlessly sat in two feet of water, and surveyed the area. His teenage eyes ogled a few mothers in their one-piece suits. As he played, his hands came across the powerful suction hole on the floor of the pool. He was surprised by the force of the suction.

He absent-mindedly tugged on the metal grate covering the suction, when he noticed Benny on the other side of the chain-link fence. He gestured towards him, and swam to the deep end to meet his friend. Arnie torpedoed down the lane, and arrived quickly, without taking a breath. As he surfaced, a familiar head stared down at him. Benny was crouching beside the edge, grinning.

"Hey Benny boy," yelled Arnie. On a whim, he grabbed Benny's shirt and yanked him into the deep end.

Benny surfaced and sputtered the heavily chlorinated water in Arnie's face.

"Way to go, asshole, this watch isn't waterproof," Benny spat, holding up a 10 dollar Seiko knock-off just above the surface. The dial had already fogged with condensation and the LCD was obscured.

"Sorry man, I couldn't resist. Besides, I was with you when we bought that piece of shit on the street. We can get another one anytime," said Arnie.

"You owe me 10 bucks," replied Benny curtly.

"Take off your shirt and stick around," said Arnie, splashing Benny and racing backwards kicking his legs.

Arnie chased Benny to the shallow end, and they splashed each other relentlessly until the lifeguard's whistle blared in their ears.

Sitting on the bottom, Arnie motioned with a shrug of his head towards a shapely woman lounging on her towel, diapered kids running around her outstretched legs. "Check out that babe," he said, flexing newly discovered hormones. He started to move a little closer when his hand lightly brushed the suction hole at the bottom. He tugged at the grate with both hands and it loosened and jumped up.

As he slithered across, he felt a searing pain in his

abdomen and buttocks. Arnie had sat on the suction hole and couldn't get up. He screamed. A hundred people went silent. He screamed again, his face frozen and white.

"I'm stuck! Help! Turn off the pool. I'm stuck!" Arnie nearly lost consciousness. Benny didn't know what to do and yelled for the lifeguard.

The lifeguard raced to Arnie's side and assessed the situation, then barged into the mechanical room and flipped the black switches down, turning off the vacuum pump. When he returned, the pool was cleared of bodies, save for Arnie, Benny, and a half dozen mothers trying to help.

As they lifted Arnie up from under his arms, the water reddened. A mother frantically dialed an ambulance, while another rushed her children away. Benny screamed and Arnie lapsed into unconsciousness. Arnie's pelvic floor had been ruptured by the suction, and his intestines were dangling out, sucked through his rectum by the pump. His small intestine had been completely eviscerated from his abdomen.

Upon arrival in the emergency room, Arnie's blood pressure was low, requiring large amounts of intravenous resuscitation. He was almost immediately transported to the operating room where a portion of his small bowel, ischemic from lack of blood flow, was resected.

Arnie made a gradual recovery. After six months, he

was nearly back to normal, despite the loss of a portion of his small intestine. He never went near water again, and developed a preference for showers and a phobia of vacuum cleaners.

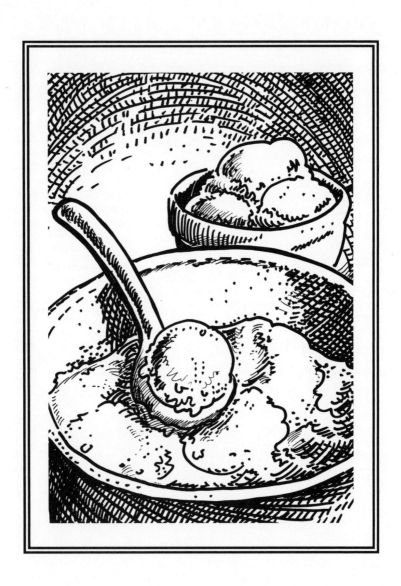

THE WOMAN
WHO SWALLOWED
A TOOTHBRUSH

There are some activities in which participants have a high likelihood of injury. Racing cars and fighting bulls are among them. Other activities are seemingly without risk, like brushing teeth in the morning. What could possibly go wrong when brushing teeth? But are routine activities truly without some risk, however small?

A 20-year-old woman was rushed to the hospital by her roommate at 10 in the morning. At the triage area, a shy, painfully slim woman, long thin hair covering her face, looked meek and uncomfortable. Unable to make eye contact with the nurse, she quietly offered up her problem with resignation and an uncharacteristically raspy voice, belying her size.

"I swallowed my toothbrush," she whispered.

"What did you say? Speak up please, it's hard to hear you when you whisper," admonished the nurse.

"I said I swallowed my toothbrush," she repeated, still barely audible.

"Now I've seen everything," thought the triage nurse, "but this isn't a pediatric center, where kids stick anything anywhere, and this is not a child."

"How did you manage to do that?" she asked with a barely concealed grin. There was little concern in her voice.

"I slipped on the bathroom floor tiles while brushing my teeth," she squeaked. "I had just stepped out of the shower and the tiles were wet. It just sort of started sliding down my throat and kept on going."

Breathing comfortably, her blood pressure fine, and only mildly tachycardic (had a rapid heart rate), she was in no real distress. The nurse guided the embarrassed patient to the acute room, and with stifled laughter explained the predicament to the emergency room doctor on call.

The clearest dictum of medicine is that a doctor has never seen it all. This doctor was wise and experienced enough to know that there was something amiss. How could a rigid six-inch object be unwillingly impaled down this young woman's throat, without her reflexively coughing it out? It seemed unlikely that a toothbrush could successfully meander down the tube-like esophagus without even a minor tear.

Despite obvious skepticism from the doctor, and subtle pressure to reconsider her story, the young woman stuck to her account of the incident.

An x-ray of the esophagus was ordered. The story unraveled immediately after the film plates were developed and the doctor reviewed them. The x-ray showed that the toothbrush was stuck with bristles pointing *upward*, toward the mouth. There was no way the toothbrush could spin 180 degrees. Either she was so confused in a morning haze, that she brushed her teeth with the wrong end, or another explanation accounted for her unfortunate predicament. The doctor showed her the x-ray, as she clung to the sheets, dwarfed by the emergency room staff that had congregated around her stretcher.

Her face was flushed. Bony fingers protruded from under her sheets. Tears rolled down her gaunt cheeks. And then the true story emerged. While attempting to induce vomiting after an early morning binge of a liter of double chocolate ice cream, she accidentally swallowed the toothbrush. The woman was suffering from bulimia. Another startling revelation was that this was the second time she had swallowed her toothbrush. The first episode was not met with such skepticism, and she escaped scrutiny by the medical staff of another emergency room.

A probe was inserted into her esophagus under anesthetic and the toothbrush was easily removed. She was referred for a voluntary psychiatric evaluation of her occult bulimia.

Bulimia is more common in women than men. It is marked by ingestion of large amounts of food, followed by an attempt to control weight by self-induced vomiting or laxative use. Although fingers are the usual method of choice to purge, anything can be used, including cutlery. Deaths have been reported from perforation of the esophagus. A toothbrush is a common bulimic tool as it resides in the bathroom, and is thus readily accessible in the most likely place to vomit.

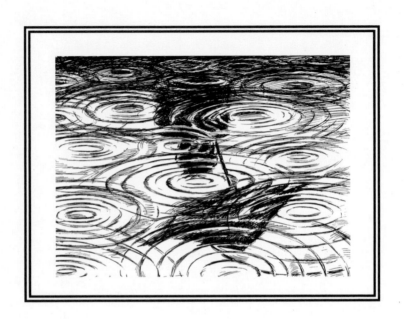

DROWNING
IN A HOSPITAL

A 72-year-old Korean man, Mr. Lee, was admitted to hospital with a large mass in his right lung.

Doctors describe smoking history according to "pack years." A pack-a-day smoker for 40 years has a 40 pack-year history. A half-pack per day for the same period translates into a 20 pack-year history. The more pack years, the greater the risk of complications. The Korean gentleman smoked three packs per day for 55 years, or 165 pack years.

A piece of the mass was obtained with a biopsy needle and the worst was confirmed: cancer. Family flocked to the hospital. Pots of Korean food were stacked high on the window sill, between old copies of Korean newspapers.

Neither his wife nor children left his room during his hospitalization. The diagnosis was explained to the man via the interpretation of his grandchildren.

Preparations were made for resection of the tumor and within a week he was wheeled into the O.R. Under the guidance of a thoracic surgeon, the right upper lobe of his lung was removed.

Mr. Lee did surprisingly well post-operatively considering the blackened state of his toxin-riddled lung tissue. Within 12 hours the endotracheal tube was removed from his throat and he was breathing on his own with minimal oxygen support. With family clustered around his bed, he was transferred from the intensive care unit to the surgical ward the following day.

Early the next morning, his daughter ran to the nursing station yelling loudly in Korean. She grabbed a nurse's arm and tugged her in the direction of her father's room. He was lying in bed in obvious respiratory distress, gasping for breath, liquid sputtering from blue lips. The nurse called a code. Within minutes, the arrest team was streaming out of the elevator, speeding their wheeled cart down the hall like a bed racing team.

The humid room was crowded with relatives shouting and crying. Nurses ushered them out and the physician evaluated the problem. He immediately placed a tube into the patient's throat and passed his vocal cords. It rested in the mainstem bronchus, just above the lungs. Clear liquid was propelled into the tube from his lungs with each breath, and was quickly removed by a slender suction catheter. The tube was connected to a pale green rubber ambu bag. The bag was rhythmically squeezed by the respiratory technician as the patient was wheeled to the intensive care unit.

Numerous diagnoses were considered by the attending physician, though none fit comfortably. It was decided he likely suffered from a combination of smoking-related lung disease (emphysema) and heart failure. Nothing else seemed to explain the copious amounts of clear liquid that poured from his mouth that heralded his sudden decline.

Mr. Lee's recovery was rapid. The breathing tube was removed early the next morning. Only a small amount of supplemental oxygen was needed, allowing transfer back to the ward later in the day.

He was moved to a private room closer to the nursing station for easier monitoring. During evening rounds, the nurse responsible for his care casually walked into his room, to find Mr. Lee face down in a blue plastic basin, spilling over with water. His head was being held down by his daughter. The nurse dropped her little containers of pills and screamed to her colleagues for assistance. Security was summoned and the daughter was placed in custody.

A Korean interpreter accompanied the police. After lengthy questioning, the events became clear. The patient was involved in a common Korean cultural practice. He was voluntarily aspirating water into his lungs to cleanse his respiratory tract, and rid himself of his tumor. The ritual was common for Mr. Lee and his family, and prior to his diagnosis, was routinely practiced in their home. His daughter had been trying to help her father, as he was weak after surgery.

On the day of his readmission to the ICU, his family recalled that while face down in the basin, he had coughed and choked on the water during his ritual and reflexively took breaths while submerged.

His readmission to the ICU was clarified, and the diagnosis modified. He suffered from a near drowning episode, miles away from any substantial body of water.

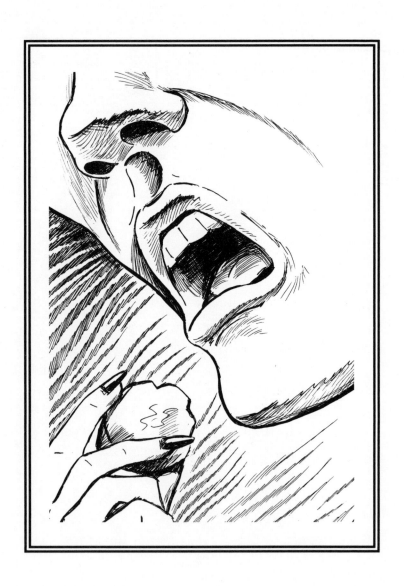

BEZOARS

A 16-year-old girl was brought to the doctor's office by her mother. After complaining of crampy abdominal pain for nearly a month, she reluctantly agreed to an evaluation.

Megan was thin and nervous, with a sallow complexion. Her long straight hair hung limply. She wore a faded gray shirt and black sweatpants. Her mother was coiffed. Her orange hair was curled like a tornado atop her head. Long earrings dangled to her shoulders. She looked like Flo, the waitress from the TV show *Alice*.

The doctor examined his young patient in the presence of her mother. He uncovered her abdomen from hips to sternum and was immediately struck by its thin and lumpy appearance. High-pitched bowel sounds met his ears as he listened over each of the four quadrants of her abdomen with his stethoscope, while Megan nervously chewed at her fingernails.

"Would you mind just leaving your arms at your sides while I examine you?" asked the doctor as his hands explored her abdomen. She uncomfortably rested her arms at her sides, in a coffin-like pose.

The doctor glided over her abdomen, pushing and kneading. A puzzled look briefly flashed and was gone. "What are these masses?" he thought. "Probably loops of stool-filled bowels."

"You can get dressed and I'll talk to you in my office," he said, and after washing his hands, left the exam room.

He sat across a small, pale wooden desk. Megan fixated on the tufts of hair leaping out of his ears like stalks of thin celery. The doctor leaned forward, hands clasped, and spoke in a monotone.

"I am concerned by your abdominal discomfort," he told Megan and her mother. "You're below your ideal body weight by 15 pounds or so, and I can feel some abnormalities in your belly. This needs further investigation."

Megan continued to nervously chew at her fingernails, grimacing as she tore out small pieces of nail leaving painful red areas near the pulp of her fingertips. Her mother gasped, and clutched her daughter's hand. Megan pulled away.

Two days later Megan found herself alone in a private room of Sick Children's Hospital. Plans were implemented for a colonoscopy. This unpleasant test involves inserting a very long flexible tube into the rectum and through the large bowel (colon). It has a camera attached to it, allowing visualization of the bowel wall by the operator, who controls the colonoscope as it passes through. Patients are understandably anesthetized with "feel good" drugs, to dull the sensation of a 10-foot tube passing in the opposite direction to the natural flow.

Megan sat in bed, fingers twisting themselves into knots. She wanted to come clean. She knew the answer to the medical question and there was no way she was going to let anyone perform this test on her.

Her doctor came into the room to review the impending procedure and answer any last-minute questions. Dressed in hospital greens, an O.R. cap covering his bald head, he spoke to his young patient.

"I need your mom here to give consent to the colonoscopy," he said to the floor. "Do you know where she is?" he asked the curtains.

Megan spoke, her high-pitched voice barely audible. "You don't need to do the test. I'll tell you what's going on."

Her thoughts spilled out. "I've been kind of changing my eating habits. If I get hungry, sometimes I don't eat food. I roll up wads of toilet paper and eat those instead. I've been doing it to lose some weight, and I think it might be causing my stomach problems."

The doctor listened, staring at her intently. Those "lumps" in Megan's abdomen were collections of rolled up toilet paper, weaving their way through her intestines. Megan had an eating disorder, and as a result her abdomen was full of bezoars, which she eventually passed.

Bezoars refer to a collection of solid undigestible material in the gastrointestinal tract. Patients with trichotilomania (hair eating compulsion) may have hair bezoars in a cast of the stomach. Elderly patients may have bezoars of undigestible plant material. This was a case of toilet paper bezoars.

Bezoars were first identified thousands of years ago. The word originated in Turkey and referred to masses found in animal stomachs, believed to have magical healing powers. Portions of the bezoar were prescribed for numerous aches and ailments.

Megan was referred to a psychiatrist for her unusual affliction.

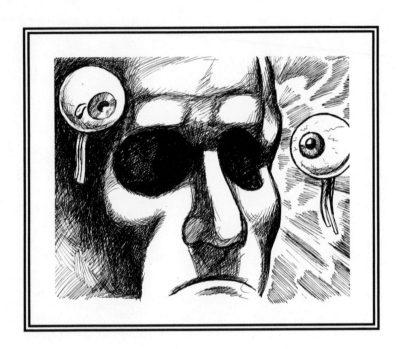

ROVING EYES

A 66-year-old Russian-speaking woman named Svetlana appeared in the emergency room complaining of bilateral eye pain. Accompanied by her family of three sons and two daughters, she spoke rapidly in Russian, gesturing wildly with her hands.

"She says her eyes hurt when she moves them," offered one of the daughters in a thick Russian accent.

On exam she obviously suffered from the ravages of thyroid-related eye disease. Her eyes protruded out of their sockets, she had a fixed wild-eyed stare with her upper eyelids barely visible, and she looked crazed and unpredictable.

The thyroid gland is a butterfly shaped organ located in

front of the trachea (in the neck). It produces thyroid hormones, which regulate the body's metabolic rate. Excessive amounts of thyroid hormone may be generated by the gland in a number of conditions. Grave's disease is an autoimmune disorder in which the body attacks the thyroid, triggering the release of large amounts of thyroid hormone. Like being under the influence of amphetamines, too much thyroid hormone (hyperthyroidism) increases heart rate and blood pressure, and causes weight loss, irritability, increased appetite, temperature intolerance, and other symptoms of a rapid metabolic rate.

Grave's disease may secondarily affect the eyes (ophthalmopathy) and cause blindness. The soft tissue behind the eyes becomes swollen with fluid, literally pushing the eyeballs forward from their protective bony enclosures. Often uncomfortable, Svetlana had been plagued by this ophthalmopathy for two years, and was prone to blurred vision, photophobia (sensitivity to light), and double vision. Embarrassed by her appearance, she rarely ventured out of her brick house.

The E.R. physician drew the curtains around her small bay in the emergency department. He tried to acquire further history, but with five children crowding around, each with a different interpretation of their mother's complaints, it was difficult.

"Tell her I want to check the pressure in her eyes, to make sure it isn't too high. That could damage her vision and would need more immediate intervention," he explained to the family. "I need to assess her risk of blindness."

A cacophony of Russian spattered the room. Gesticulating and yelling, six voices struggled to be heard. After a few minutes the din died down, and the doctor brought out a small device to measure the pressure within the eyes.

"Ask her to lie down please," he began. "Tell her I am going to rest the device on each eye. It will be painless and quick."

She appeared to understand. The room was calm as he gently placed the measuring device on her eye, and then it happened.

Svetlana sneezed, and as she did, her eyes leapt out of their sockets and dangled over her cheeks. Her eyes were attached at the center to the white cord-like optic nerve, and surrounded by the extra-ocular muscles. These muscles attach to the eyes like thick parachute strings, guiding movement in all directions. The blue eyes swung from side to side as she turned her head. A perfect and inexpensive Halloween costume.

She screamed in pain, two children fainted in terror, and the others yelled loudly, imploring the doctor to do something. Faced with a sneezing induced bilateral enucleation, he knew there was only one thing he could do: pop the eyes back in. Without hesitation, he carefully donned a pair of sterile surgical gloves. Gently grasping her eyeballs one at a time to howls of protest, he plunked them back into their sockets like pegs in a hole.

She gazed at the doctor (with both eyes). He was unsure whether she was about to attack as she stared through him. She quietly thanked him (in Russian).

"That happens all the time doctor," explained the youngest daughter. "Now, what can we do about her pain?"

With that the young doctor left the room and called the ophthalmology service to come down to the E.R. and take a look.

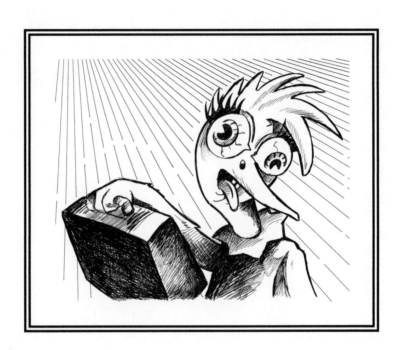

WOODY
WOODPECKER'S
A COMMUNIST

"Woody Woodpecker's a communist, Woody Woodpecker's a communist . . ." The chant filled the halls of the emergency department, drowning the usual noises of illness and technology. None of the staff stopped what they were doing or turned to stare. Just another loonie brought in by the cops. Patients and their relatives were more interested in the scene, not used to the daily machinations of a busy urban emergency room. "Kill the brussel sprouts!" he screamed.

Lying face down on a stretcher, arms handcuffed to the railings, feet restrained by thick leather straps, and held down by four burly policemen was a man in a well-tailored business suit. It was probably smaller than when it first came off the rack, as the man was soaking wet. Puddles of water formed around his stretcher like a moat. He twisted left and right, the bulk of him immobilized, glued to the stretcher.

Dangling from his arm and attached to his wrist by another set of handcuffs of his own was a reinforced smooth, silver, steel briefcase. It was protected by a 10-digit locking mechanism.

"You're up, Kevin," the nurse said to the emerg doctor, as she walked away from the patient, rolling her eyes as she passed. The doctor slowly moved over to the scene, shoulders sagging, feet dragging. Psych cases were not his favorite. He was anticipating a quick check and even quicker referral to the psychiatry service.

A cursory exam disclosed nothing physically wrong. The man was lean, fit, and wet. His hair was short and plastered to his head. His nails were well manicured and his leather shoes expensive, Italian, and ruined. His wallet identified him as Gerhardt, 32 years old and a German citizen. He had $2,000 in cash and a dozen credit cards. His address was listed as a downtown penthouse condo. His coat pocket housed several large and soggy cigars.

"Eat the pillow Woody," he yelled. "Eat the pillow." His face was ruddy and swollen, his lips bruised. A small river of blood slowly cascaded from the corner of his mouth, which housed perfectly straight and white teeth, except for one missing incisor.

Gerhardt was a banker. While strolling down the waterfront minding his own business, a voice directed him to jump to his death over the Niagara Falls. Seizing the opportunity, he deduced that the fastest route to the Niagara Falls was Lake Ontario, conveniently located a mere 50 yards away. He took off at a gallop and leapt in.

The police marine unit, alerted to the jump by a large crowd of pedestrians, boated into action and found Gerhardt swimming fully clothed toward the middle of Lake Ontario, dragging his heavy steel briefcase cuffed to his wrist. Though a strong swimmer, he appeared to be tiring.

Unwilling to be rescued, he fought off the police charge doggedly. Four members of the marine unit were obligated to jump into the balmy July waters and "rescue" the unwilling banker. They dropped him off at the hospital. Fearing for their safety from an obviously crazed German banker in expensive clothing, the bomb disposal unit was called in to investigate the suitcase. Looking like members of a football team in the emergency room, they were unable to penetrate the thick steel case with their equipment.

They contemplated the only two options available to a bomb unit: open or destroy? They elected to open it, though they first cut through the chain connecting it to Gerhardt.

"Eleven monkeys are too many," advised Gerhardt, oblivious to the drama around him.

Taking the briefcase gingerly to a thick oval bomb-proof drum, one brave member was directed to pick the lock. The event transpired in the parking lot of the emergency room, though one can imagine that this would offer no advantage to the hapless team member if the case truly housed explosives.

Within the steel walls of the small rectangular case was $26 million in negotiable bonds, stolen from the bank vault that morning. Gerhardt had developed an acute psychotic episode and his hallucinations were guiding him in many directions.

The doctor strolled away from the scene and put in a call to psychiatry, as he knew he would from the outset. He shook his head in disappointment, wondering what he would have done had he got his hands on the suitcase first.

"The Arctic will rule you," yelled Gerhardt helpfully, as a needle of anti-psychotic medication was rammed into his buttocks.

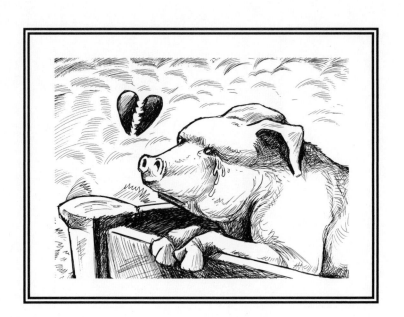

ZOOPHILIA

Abdominal pain is a common presenting complaint in the emergency room. At any moment in the E.R. triage room, at least one patient will drag himself in, bent over from severe and unrelenting pain. There are causes too numerous to list for abdo pain. Some are serious and need immediate life-saving surgery, while others are benign and self-limiting.

A 58-year-old farmer with abdominal pain drove himself to the hospital. It took him three hours of bone-jarring driving over unpaved roads to get from his remote farm to the emergency department. His blood pressure was dangerously low and his heart rate was elevated. The triage nurse directed the orderly to wheel Jed into the acute room immediately. He was quickly set upon by a team of nurses and doctors. Intravenous lines were started, and x-rays ordered. He began to lapse out of consciousness.

A tough and independent character, he waited 14 hours before deciding the pain was not going to spontaneously resolve. His wife, Clara, had finally cajoled him into making an appearance at hospital, though he insisted on driving.

Outside the acute room, Clara told one of the nurses the story. "He was out back in the barn for the whole day," she began. "When he came in for supper, he was grimacing, and seemed to have trouble getting in through the kitchen door. I asked him what was wrong, but he just grabbed onto the counter, made his way to the table and didn't say nothin'. I made his favorite supper, but he couldn't take a bite. I had to help him from the table into the parlor, and he finally told me Nelle, one of our horses, had kicked him in the gut. I guess he didn't want to say nothin' cuz I'd start gettin' on him about lettin' the workers do some of the labor. But Jed loves animals."

Jed's condition was deteriorating. "Open up his IV lines, and let's start some dopamine, his pressure is dropping," shouted the emerg doc. "He's got an acute abdomen. Let's prep him and get him to the operating room."

Jed's wife signed the procedure consent form, since Jed was no longer alert. He was rushed to the operating room and cut open. His abdomen was full of stool and the thin surgical masks were unhelpful in combating the feculent aroma. The operating room staff moaned and groaned with each inhalation. The surgeon flushed the peritoneal cavity with saline to cleanse his organs of the feces. He explored the sausage-like intestines and located a ragged tear in the rectum.

The intestines are a long tube full of waste. There can never be a compromise of the lining (called the mucosa) or, as in Jed's case, feces will leak out and cause bacterial peritonitis. Before the dawn of antibiotics, peritonitis was uniformly fatal. Houdini died from peritonitis in 1926. Had antibiotics been available, his ailment would have been quickly and easily cured.

Jed was sewn up and he quickly improved. Days later, despite cajoling and support, he refused to disclose how he tore his rectum. The surgeons knew something was shoved up there, but had no idea what. The rectum does not spontaneously tear. Clara was oblivious to the dilemma, and slept peacefully by her husband's side. Eventually a psychiatrist was consulted, and Jed confessed to the source of his adventure.

Jed had a girlfriend, though not in the conventional sense of the word. Bollah, the prize boar, was more than just a state fair winner. It turns out Bollah was part of Jed's daytime and nocturnal barnyard trysts. Jed was partaking in sexual intercourse with a boar.

A boar's penis is corkscrew shaped, and twists into a point. The right side is stronger than the left, and as the muscles contract and relax, the penis twists back and forth like a screw. It latches onto the ridges of the sow's vagina before rapidly twisting and culminating in payload delivery. The boar's penis tore Jed's rectum.

Jed admitted to multiple sexual partners, but refused to implicate other members of his menagerie. The medical staff did not break patient confidentiality and inform his wife of his animal escapades. Clara took him home two weeks after admission, seemingly oblivious to the competition.

Zoophilia or bestiality is much more common than reported. Most cases end without the need for medical intervention.

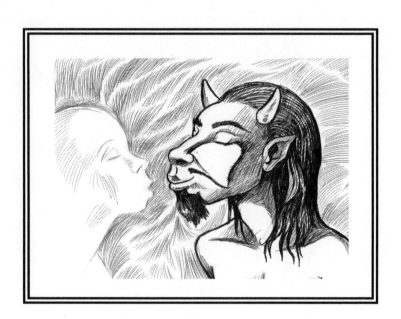

INSATIABLE

A 22-year-old man was evaluated by a psychiatrist as part of a court order. He had been arrested for frotteurism, sexual satisfaction obtained by rubbing against unwilling participants. Frotteurism is practiced on public transportation and at sporting events and other locations characterized by close contact in enclosed spaces. "Howard" was caught between periods of a professional hockey game, rubbing up against a young woman attending with her father. He was so excited by the act, he had an orgasm. Security guards saved him from getting his lights punched out, rushing to his aid as he was set upon by the father and other irate hockey fans.

The psychiatrist looked like a bald version of Santa Claus. Elderly and rotund, he wore a drab brown three-piece suit. A pocket watch crossed over his generous abdomen, and thick glasses magnified his eyeballs. He was squished into a leather arm chair two sizes too small for his frame. Howard had been granted bail, on condition that he attend counseling prior to his court date. He entered the doctor's office unaccompanied, unshaven, and dressed in a track suit. He was motioned to a simple cushioned chair in the office.

"You know why you're here Howard," the psychiatrist stated. "Tell me about yourself."

"I'm horny as hell every waking moment," Howard began, and his story quickly unfolded.

Howard was married to a woman nearly twice his age. They had sexual intercourse three times a day and he mastur-bated an additional four times per day. His preference was more frequent consensual sex; however he and his wife agreed to thrice daily intercourse as a compromise. His masturbation was peppered with fantasies of sado-masochism, and included inflatable dolls, a vacuum, and liberal visual aids in the form of videos and magazines. He had subscriptions to nearly a dozen pornographic monthlies.

He had "wet dreams" many times a week. A frequent and recurrent dream involved him being shrunk to four inches in height. He would then travel in a condom ship, exploring the vaginas of women he knew. Howard had the ability to reach an orgasm simply by exploring his fantasies, without the need for tactile stimulation.

His sexual fantasies dated back to his earliest memories. He would frequently excuse himself from class to masturbate in the washroom. He was always in relationships with classmates during high school. They usually terminated because of his insatiable sexual needs.

His father died suddenly when Howard was six years old. Thereafter he developed a very close relationship with his mother, and periodically slept in her bed until he was 16 years old. He also regressed, and started to suck his thumb and wet his bed. Howard was an excellent student and regular church-goer.

While in university, Howard met his wife. They were engaged and married within a year. He described his wife as being mature, understanding, and capable, "exactly like my mother."

Howard continued to fantasize about nearly every woman he knew including friends, acquaintances, and those he simply passed on the street. He began affairs with co-workers and neighbors soon after his marriage and frequented prostitutes at least twice a week.

He had never been charged with deviant sexual behavior prior to his arrest, though admitted he enjoyed voyeurism around his apartment complex and often attended sporting events to grope unsuspecting women.

Howard was aware that his sexual urges were excessive (known as satyriasis in males, nymphomania in females), but was more concerned about being caught. He attended sessions with the good doctor for months. After intensive psychotherapy, absolutely no progress was made. His sexual appetite remained elevated and the court sentenced him to six months' probation.

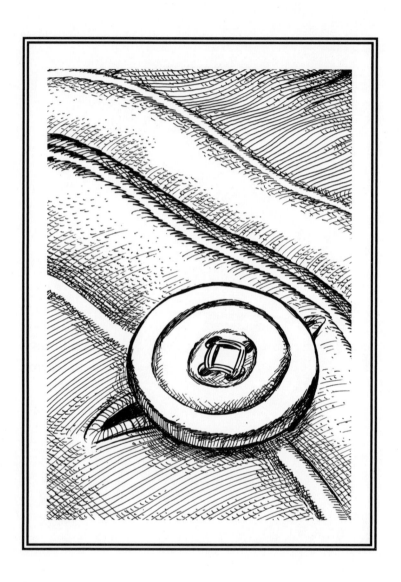

ATYPICAL CHEST PAIN

A 40-year-old woman presented to a cardiologist for a second opinion. She had a one-year history of sharp left-sided chest pain exacerbated by movement. She had no history of smoking, diabetes, high blood pressure, or cholesterol abnormalities.

Her family practitioner was unable to find a cause and referred her to a cardiologist. His investigations included a normal stress test and cardiac ultrasound, after which he dismissed her complaints as non-cardiac and sent her back to the GP. He concluded her discomfort was likely musculo-skeletal in origin and prescribed anti-inflammatories with negligible benefit. She insisted something was wrong with her and demanded a second opinion.

The second cardiologist reviewed the findings and came to the same conclusion as the first, namely that the pain was non-cardiac in origin. Unconvinced, she returned to her family doctor.

He appeared annoyed when he entered the small exam room and met her eyes. "So I assume you are still having pain?" he asked curtly.

"I'm not sure what to do. The pain is continuing. It's not too severe but I'm really bothered by it because I know something is wrong. Is there anything else you can do or anywhere else to send me?" she lamented, tears in her eyes.

"Look," began her doctor. "It's obviously not your heart, and it's been there for a year already. Whatever it is, isn't going to kill you. I think you should just live with it. Let me give you a stronger painkiller."

He produced a rectangular prescription pad from his lab coat pocket and scribbled a quick script for codeine. He handed it to her, and turned to leave.

Despondent, she returned home. Though her pain was troubling, she found herself more troubled by her conviction something was wrong. She decided to go to the local emergency department.

Arriving at 8 p.m., the E.R. was a zoo. She calmly relayed her story to the triage nurse. Obviously comfortable and in no distress, she waited four hours before finally seeing a doctor. He was young, tired, and had a harried look. He barely glanced up from her chart as he entered the room and introduced himself.

"I'm Doctor Wright," he began. "It says here you have some chest pain?"

She began to cry as her story spilled out. "The pain isn't severe but it won't go away. Every time I take a deep breath or cough it gets a bit worse, especially if I'm on my left side."

On exam, her blood pressure, heart rate, respiratory rate, and cardiorespiratory exams were completely normal. Dr. Wright tried to reassure his young patient. "It really doesn't sound like an issue. I think you should go home and I am sure it will get better soon. I'll let the nurse know you're ready to head out."

"No," she said defiantly. "There's something wrong and you have to find out what. Order a chest x-ray." Taken aback, Dr. Wright became defensive. "Look, you've been investigated thoroughly. It's time to accept your pain has no organic basis."

"The chest x-ray. Just order one and I'll be on my way. I'm not leaving until you help. Call security if you want." She stared him down.

Reluctant and defeated, he sighed, left the cubicle, and ordered a lateral and postero-anterior (two views) chest x-ray. It was too late to fight and he wanted this wacko out of his hair. "Why always on my shift?" he thought.

Just before going for his 2 a.m. coffee, Dr. Wright passed by the radiology resident on call. "Ronald, come here," said the resident. "I was just gonna get you. Take a look at the x-ray on room 6." He slipped the films on the view box and turned on the back light. Dr. Wright no longer needed the coffee. His heart raced. His jaw opened. A thin sliver shone back at him from the chest x-ray, seemingly embedded in the woman's heart.

He raced back to his patient. He was effusive and obsequious. He stared at the floor, his shoes, the curtains, everywhere but her face. "There seems to be an irregularity on your chest x-ray."

She knew it. She was calm and didn't get angry. She just wanted answers.

"I'd like to get a CAT scan. We're not sure what it is, but it looks like a long needle or something."

The CAT scan confirmed his suspicion. Embedded in the outer lining of the heart (the pericardium), and abutting the main chamber of the heart, was a sewing needle.

When questioned further, she vaguely recalled falling asleep on the couch a year previously while sewing a button on her son's baseball uniform. She had awoken short of breath with sharp chest pain, but the sensation had passed and she thought little of it, unable to sort out the reason for her symptoms.

She was admitted to hospital. The following day, a cardiothoracic surgeon was called. He introduced a thorascope into her chest cavity and under visual guidance, retrieved the offending sewing needle. Her recovery was uncomplicated and she was sent home the following day. She switched family doctors and sent a copy of her discharge summary to all of her previous physicians. None contacted her, and none offered an apology.

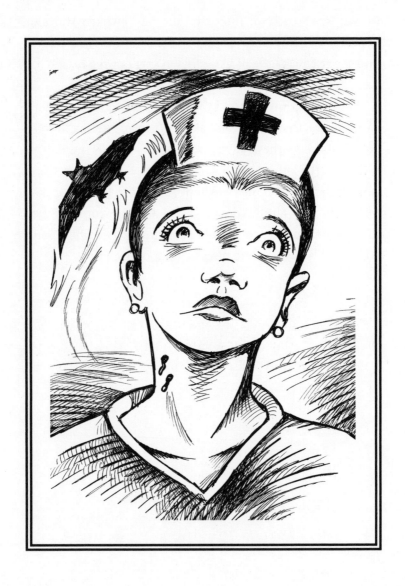

A RARE CAUSE
OF ANEMIA

A 32-year-old nurse was admitted to hospital with anemia.
Her history included unexplained anemia eight years
previously during the third trimester of her third pregnancy. She required a transfusion of three units of red
blood cells.

The bloodstream is a liquid highway, a lengthy,
constantly moving supply route for the body. Oxygen is
necessary for the proper function of all cells. It dissolves in
blood, but in miniscule amounts compared to that transported by red blood cells (RBCs). The oxygen travels in red
blood cells bound to a special protein structure called
hemoglobin. Oxygen requires iron to bind to hemoglobin.

This is why dietary iron is necessary to form blood cells capable of binding and transporting oxygen.

Hemoglobin measurements are a direct reflection of how many red blood cells there are, and indicate the blood's oxygen carrying capacity. Anemic patients have low hemoglobin levels. Less fuel tires the body and causes fatigue and breathlessness.

Anemia is caused by many conditions. The most obvious is blood loss. Blood loss may be occult, making it difficult to identify. Blood may slowly seep from somewhere in the gastrointestinal tract, such as a gastric or duodenal ulcer. Blood may quietly flow from polyps or tumors in the colon, like lava from a volcano. It may trickle from the bladder or kidney. The most common cause of anemia in a young woman is heavy menstruation. Epistaxis, the medical term for nosebleeds, is an occasional cause of anemia. Other types of blood loss are called melena, hematemesis, hematochezia, hemoptysis, menorhaggia, and hematuria.

The other end of the anemia puzzle is production. Low dietary intake or poor gastric absorption of iron, vitamin B12, or folate will inhibit red blood cell production and cause anemia. The bone marrow, site of red blood cell production, may be poisoned by many toxins. Medications may rarely interfere with red blood cell production. The bone marrow may be invaded by tumors that interfere with RBC production.

Finally, red blood cells might be produced normally, but may be destroyed within the bloodstream. This destruction is called hemolysis. It is often autoimmune, meaning the body produces antibodies that destroy the RBCs.

When a patient presents to the doctor with anemia, a history, physical exam, and investigations almost always identify the cause. Perhaps there is a drug the patient is taking, or they report blood loss from some orifice.

Alcoholics are often vitamin deficient. Alcohol can cause stomach inflammation and ulcers. A history of excessive use may be the only clue needed. A long tube (a gastro-scope) can be introduced into the stomach to directly visualize an ulcer. A tube may also go up the other end (a colonoscope) to look for tumors and ulcers. Another tube (this time a cystoscope) investigates bladder tumors.

If no source of blood loss can be identified, simple blood tests (more blood loss!) can be performed to diagnose hemolysis. Finally, the bone marrow may be sampled with a biopsy. A large hollow needle is inserted into the hip bone and a core of bone is twisted and yanked out using both hands, like pulling a tooth. The sample is reviewed under a microscope to see if enough cells are present, and search for an infiltrating cancer.

The nurse was tired. Her fatigue began six months previously and was progressing. She was on disability, unable to carry out her nursing duties. A checklist of questions was posed, but the answers failed to identify a source of blood loss. She was not taking any medications such as aspirin that could cause bleeding, denied illicit drug use, and did not drink excessively. On exam, her complexion was monstrously pale. The whites of her eyes (conjunctivae) were very white. Her blood pressure was normal and she was mildly tachycardic with a heart rate of 110 beats per minute. There was no abnormal collection of lymph nodes and no mass when poked and prodded. Her hemoglobin level was 60 (normal 120–140). Despite numerous diagnostic tests, no abnormalities were visualized.

After a million dollar work-up, a bone marrow aspiration and biopsy were performed. When reviewed by the pathologist, he reported normal amounts of iron and hypercellularity with excessive reticulocytes.

When blood cells are made in the bone marrow, there are many stages of production towards maturity. If huge numbers of soldiers are killed on the battlefield, new less experienced recruits are forced onto the frontlines. RBCS work the same way. If the normal mature cells disappear, either by bleeding or destruction, immature forms proliferate and are sent into the bloodstream early. These cells are anatomically distinct from normal blood cells and called reticulocytes.

The woman's reticulocyte count narrowed down the cause. Blood loss must be the answer. But despite a complete search, no blood loss could be identified. Special tagged red blood cells were injected in search of a microleak, with no result. Hemoglobin may be genetically abnormal (sickle cell disease, thalassemia). This was tested and excluded. After a transfusion of two units of blood she felt well enough to leave hospital.

Two months later the nurse presented to another hospital with the same problem. The same tests were performed, again with no result. She was transfused again and discharged. Three months after that, a third hospital admitted her. Same story, same result. Within a year, she was admitted four times to four different hospitals.

An annual international hematology conference was convening in Lausanne, Switzerland. It was an opportunity for research to be shared amongst leading experts. During an evening party, a group of old friends, all hematologists from the same state, enjoyed a meal in the formal dining room. Drinks flowed with the conversation.

"I had this wild case last month," began one of them. "A young nurse came in with a hemoglobin of 60. Couldn't find a cause. Couldn't think of any more bloody tests, I mean we went through all of her. Nothing."

Silence. Three of the six hematologists sat forward, and each relayed the same story. She had come to each of their hospitals with the same problem, and within a minute they all came to the same conclusion. By the end of the evening, they agreed that one of their members would arrange a follow-up in his clinic and a plan was hatched.

Within a month, the young pale nurse was seen in the clinic, willing and unknowing. Not surprisingly, her hemo-globin was 64, and admission was recommended, which she grudgingly accepted.

A videocamera was hidden in her room and the mode of blood loss confirmed. The doctors, sitting around that circular table in Switzerland half-drunk, understood that for every medical question there is an answer, not to be confused with "for every medical problem there is a solu-tion." There are a finite number of explanations for blood loss, numerous but finite.

This 32-year-old woman was responsible for her own blood loss. The cameras caught her bleeding herself with a simple intravenous needle. She took small amounts of her own blood, and instead of donating it, dumped it down the toilet.

When confronted, she initially denied the accusations, but became quiet and withdrawn when faced with the video evidence. A psychiatrist was consulted and the nurse was "sectioned," involuntarily committed to hospital. The psychiatrist assessed her to be a danger to herself. Two months after discharge she was hit by a bus and died of massive blood loss.

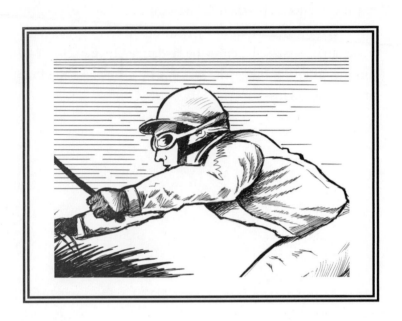

JOCKEYING FOR POSITION

A jockey was thrown from his horse. The 5'2", 102-pound jockey was riding a 1,200-pound horse at 32 miles an hour. The field of eight horses and riders was tight on the last turn of a half-mile race at the local track. Squeezed against the siderail, the horse's front legs buckled. The snap of his foreleg bones echoed through the grandstands. The jockey weightlessly tumbled forward. What seemed like an hour of flight lasted under two seconds. He loudly thumped on the soft dirt, landing on his back. His last recollection was fear. The horse, called Miles To Go, was noisier as he landed on the jockey, sumersaulting head over tail. The horse's neck was broken, and the jockey broke limbs and ribs.

The jockey's neck was immobilized with a spinal collar and he was transported by helicopter to a level one trauma center. Chest tubes were inserted by the trauma team and copious streams of blood drained from his chest. In shock, he was intubated by the anesthetist for airway control.

Blood products poured into him through intravenous lines. Large amounts of packed red blood cells, platelets, and fresh frozen plasma were infused. His pelvis, both femurs, humeris, fibulas, tibias, and eight ribs were fractured. A smooth glistening stick of bone, jagged and red, poked through his knee. One kidney was split in half, his spleen ruptured, and his liver lacerated. Despite a concussion, there was no evidence of intracerebral hemorrhaging.

"I don't think this guy is going to make it," said the trauma surgeon. "This kind of injury is just too severe. Let's get ortho, general surgery, urology, neurosurg, and a chaplain down here."

With massive trauma, the kidneys shut down in a survival mode. Urine production slows to a crawl, as the kidneys are not adequately perfused with blood. More urine production means less liquid in the bloodstream. When faced with blood loss, the body must retain as much fluid as possible in order to stave off death.

The jockey, from the moment he arrived in the emergency room and despite massive blood loss, peed like a racehorse. He was producing 300 milliliters of dilute urine per hour. Normal production is 40–60 per hour. With the urine came potassium, and his serum potassium level was dangerously low. This was contrary to normal physiology. Blood loss causes oliguria (low urine volume) not polyuria.

More than 100 units of blood products were transfused in the first 24 hours of his arrival at the hospital. He used up most of the blood bank's supply. For days the surgeons worked. The bones were set, the organs stitched. Against overwhelming odds, he survived day to day, in critical condition. He continued to pour out liters and liters of urine as his blood pressure hovered around undetectable levels. After a few days his urine output normalized. No cause for the polyuria was identifed by the nephrologist (kidney specialist).

"There is one last possibility," said the astute clinician. He conferred with the gaggle of horse riders jockeying for position in a vigil around the bedside and confirmed his suspicions.

A common pre-race practice in the horse racing world is the use of Lasix (also called furosemide), a powerful diuretic. Lasix interferes with the absorption of sodium in the renal tubules. As sodium passes unabsorbed through these porous tunnels, water is an obligatory follower. The jockey took a huge dose of Lasix hours before the race to lighten himself for the journey by peeing out huge amounts of urine. It worked too late and too long. Excessive doses of Lasix cause ringing in the ears (tinnitus), muscle cramps, lightheadedness, and balance difficulties. Review of a video of the race showed the jockey was clearly not in control of his horse during the accident, which may have contributed to his downfall. Perhaps his bladder was full or his excessive urine production before the race made him lightheaded.

He miraculously survived, and after six months of rehabilitation he was able to walk with the use of two canes. He never rode a horse again.

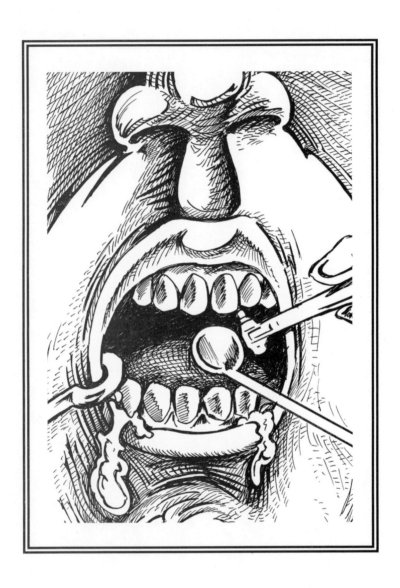

DENTAL
COMPLICATIONS

A 38-year-old dentist came to the emergency room with progressive numbness of his hands and feet over the past month.

"It started about four weeks ago," the dentist told the doctor. "First my toes, then my calves and thighs were affected. Lately, I'm having trouble feeling my fingers and hands. It's all numb."

"Any other symptoms?" asked the doctor.

"Well," he began, "I've been constipated and I'm having trouble controlling my urine. It's getting so I can't work."

On exam, he was a pleasant but anxious fellow. The

emergency room physician performed a number of neuro-logic maneuvers. He found that the dentist had no sensation below his calves and forearms when jabbed with the dulled tip of a safety pin. He had a wide-based gait, and seemed unable to easily stand upright. A Romberg's sign was positive. In this test the patient is asked to stand with feet together and arms outstretched. He is then instructed to close his eyes. In a normal person, balance is main-tained. The dentist fell backwards into the waiting arms of the doctor. His job was done. Now that a neurologic abnor-mality was found, the emergency room was far too busy to probe further. He had to move on to the next case. Neurology was consulted.

Neurology is the study of brain, spinal cord (called the central nervous system), and nerve disorders. It has often been described as a branch of medicine that can pinpoint a neurological condition from subtle exam findings with an unparalleled exactness. Unfortunately, the description is precise but the treatment options are nearly absent.

The chief neurologist wandered down to the emergency room late in the afternoon, trailed by an imprinted group of medical students and junior doctors. Dr. Schwann was a tall and thin elderly man, with a perfect helmet of gray hair. He wore a striped dress shirt with polka-dot tie, had a predilection for purple slacks, and spoke with a soft

English accent. Single with no children, he never smiled. He was married to his work. A glance and raised eyebrow was all that was required to silence his charges. Dr. Schwann was a man of control.

He entered the cubicle, temporary housing for the neuropathic dentist, and in a clear monotone rattled off a slew of questions. Medical history, surgical history, medications, habits, family history, diet. On and on he questioned the dentist, an audience of six watching.

Dr. Schwann proceeded to examine the patient. With the deftness of decades of experience, he completed the full neurologic exam in 12½ minutes.

He finished the exam, and pronounced the diagnosis: "You have subacute combined degeneration of the spinal cord." With a brief flourish, he exited the cubicle, and as he did, barked orders to the trailing junior resident. "Admit him, get a B12 level, folate, antibodies to parietal cells and intrinsic factor, Schilling test, and syphilis screen. Check him for HIV, EBV, and CMV. Get TFTS, an ESR, ANA, RF, and spinal cord MRI."

Dumbfounded, the confused dentist was admitted to the neurology ward, its main denizens partly functioning stroke patients. The resident spent an hour apologizing for the brusqueness of Dr. Schwann, and explained that there was a serious spinal cord problem.

The MRI confirmed diffuse injury to portions of the spinal cord. All lab tests were normal, aside from very low levels of vitamin B12.

"Good news," smiled the resident. "It seems you have vitamin B12 deficiency. It's easily treatable with simple oral supplements, but we can't figure out the cause. Are you sure your diet is normal?"

Before the dentist had a chance to respond, the imposing figure of Dr. Schwann appeared at the threshold of the room. He stood by the side of the hospital bed. "You have vitamin B12 deficiency. I have had the opportunity to review your test results. Only one possibility exists. You are a nitrous oxide abuser. I suggest you cease this practice." He turned and left without waiting for a response.

"How the hell did he know that?" asked the incredulous dentist.

"You mean he's right?" inquired the resident. "You inhale the nitrous oxide in your dental office?"

"It started a few years ago," explained the dentist. "It's called nanging. I got hooked on the high. I go through loads of the stuff. We used to have nitrous parties at the office, but we got into some legal difficulties with a few of the assistants and had to pay settlements."

Nitrous oxide renders vitamin B12 inactive by affecting the cobalt atom on the vitamin. Vitamin B12 is involved in the integrity of myelin, a component of neurologic tissue in the spinal cord. Without B12, the myelin doesn't work, and without myelin, specific areas of spinal cord function are impaired causing numbness and gait disturbances. Nanging often afflicts medical staff, but has become an increasingly frequent source of recreational drug abuse.

Dr. Schwann, with the wisdom of a lengthy medical career, had seen such cases before, and quickly deduced the diagnosis from the laboratory investigations. The dentist continued nanging, but made sure to take megadoses of vitamin B12 supplements.

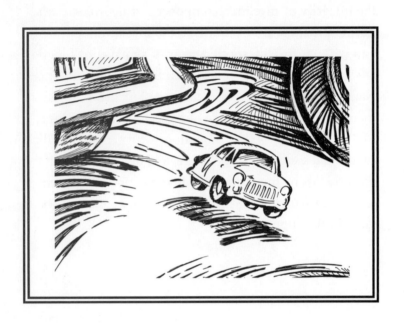

MUSCLE CAR

A 42-year-old man, 1,200 miles from home, drove himself to hospital complaining of diffuse muscle aches (myalgia) associated with a brownish hue to his urine. A salesman, he was on his way to a conference, and eagerly anticipated a meeting with his business associate. Hoping to drive through the night, he had been on the highways for nearly 20 hours, stopping briefly for gas and caffeine.

He had no previous medical history, was on no medications, and saw his physician for yearly check-ups. About 19 hours into his long journey, he began to feel pain in his thighs, buttocks, and lower back. It progressed in severity and he elected to stop at a Holiday Inn, disappointed that he was only 100 miles from his destination. Fatigued from the drive, he quickly fell asleep. He awoke periodically with aches and pains, and in the morning the myalgias were still present. He slept eight hours but felt more fatigued than ever. "It must be the flu," he thought.

He voided, and was shocked to see brown liquid stream into the toilet. He called his business associate, informed her he would be late for their rendezvous, and drove to the hospital.

He waited a few hours in the emergency room before a young doctor called him to an examining room. She quickly took a history. His vital signs were normal and he had diffuse muscle aches on palpation.

"I'm really not sure why your muscles hurt," she explained unhelpfully, "but let's do a few simple blood tests. I'm not happy with this brown urine story."

"What do you mean you're not happy?" he asked.

"Urine is only made in one color," she responded. "If a patient tells me it's anything but yellow, that's a reason to do a few tests. We'll check your blood and urine, it won't take long. Just a couple of hours. I'll still be on shift and I promise to talk to you about the results." With that she turned on her heels, handed the chart to a nurse, and disappeared from view.

A large nurse rumbled in 10 minutes later, a small bag

of supplies in her hand. She was all business. "Let's get those samples the doctor ordered," she said.

She tied a rubber tourniquet around his left upper arm. "Squeeze your fist, you'll just feel a little prick."

"That's what I tell my wife," he quipped. She didn't say anything as the bevel stung him. Purple blood spilled into the vacutainer bottle, sucked in by the vacuum. He hated getting poked with needles.

"Here's a cup. Fill it," she instructed.

"With what?" he joked. She didn't answer and left the room.

He didn't feel a need to pee. He tossed the clear plastic bottle with the pink top from hand to hand and decided to give it a go. It was tough, but he was able to shoot 20 milliliters of cloudy brown urine into the cup. He screwed on the top, and took the bottle to the nurse. His legs ached.

An hour later, the young doctor appeared. This time she took a seat. He read concern on her face.

"You've got a problem," she started.

"Great," he thought. "I've got a problem."

"It seems your kidneys have shut down. You're in acute renal failure."

"That's not possible," he said. "What do you mean renal failure? I'm healthy. How can my kidneys just shut down?"

"I don't know for sure," she offered. "There are a lot of

possibilities and it's a bit beyond my expertise. Your urea and creatinine are high. They're sort of like poisons the body makes as it functions, like toxic by-products. Anyways, yours are too high, which means the kidneys are not excreting them like they should. Your potassium is over six, so the kidneys aren't excreting that either. You need to be prepared for hemodialysis."

"Dialysis? It was just some muscle aches and brown urine, what are you talking about?" he said desperately.

"Look, you need to call your family. I've got a call in for the nephrologist. You need admission now, and he'll have to put in a dialysis catheter, either in your neck or groin."

He didn't know what to say. Gripped by fear and dread, he was certain he was going to die. He decided not to call his wife, but told his business partner that something came up and he would not be able to meet for dinner.

A half an hour later, the kidney specialist appeared, eager to get started. He was young, a bit too enthusiastic, and had a habit of raising his eyebrows at the end of every sentence. His stutter was barely perceptible. A tic opened and closed his left eye every 10 seconds or so and, like the stuttering, was beyond his control. He wore white sneakers with three narrow blue stripes, and old jeans. His white button-down shirt was clean and pressed. The patient's first thought was, "This guy must still live with his mother."

He introduced himself. "Hi, I'm Doctor P-P-Peabody. D-D-Dr. Ramones told me about you. I need to ask you the s-s-same questions she did."

He went through all the same questions, and was particularly interested in the car trip.

"S-S-So you're saying you were in the car for 19 hours? What kind of c-c-car?"

"Toyota Echo. What the hell's the difference?" he intoned.

"Well, your blood test shows a CK level of 52,000. CK stands for creatine kinase. It's what we see in the bloodstream when muscles are d-d-damaged. This is wh-wh-what caused your kidney failure. It's t-t-toxic to the kidneys in large amounts. Muscle damage like this is called rhabdomyolysis. It h-h-happens when people are confined in one space for long periods or can't move for some reason. It's seen a lot in s-s-survivors of earthquakes, or in al-al-alcoholics who are unconscious for a long time. Your kidney failure is from high levels of CK from r-r-rhabdomyolysis."

"This is Greek to me Doc, I'm just a salesman. What the hell caused it?"

"Your car," he replied. "You stayed in a little c-c-compact car for almost 24 hours. Your muscles were crushed by the pressure of just sitting, immobilized for long periods of time. High levels of m-m-myoglobin, another product of muscle damage, turn the urine brown. You need dialysis, but hopefully just for the short term."

He was rehydrated with huge volumes of intravenous saline and, after two uncomfortable weeks hooked up to the hemo machine thrice weekly, was released from hospital. His wife never came to visit, and he convalesced in the arms of his business associate.

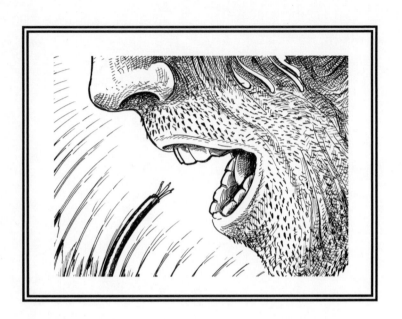

BAD HABITS

A 49-year-old electrician complained of persistent abdominal pain and constipation. He was at the end of his rope. After numerous hospital admissions, he had been recently discharged yet again without a diagnosis. The pain had begun four months earlier. It was constant and diffuse, throughout the abdomen.

During his most recent admission to a large community hospital, he had undergone a potpourri of invasive tests, including a colonoscopy, gastroscopy, and ultimately, an exploratory laporotomy.

A colonoscopy allows a gastroenterologist to view the inside of the intestines with a long flexible black tube called a colonoscope. It resembles an 18-foot snake, and has a camera at the end. As it passes through the intestine, air is flushed in to expand the walls of the "tunnel" making it easier to see if there are any tumors, polyps, ulcers, or other sources of bleeding and discomfort.

As those fortunate enough to have had a long rubber tube thrust up their rear ends will confirm, the worst part of the test is not the procedure itself. An intravenous cocktail of valium and its relatives is so calming, most wouldn't care if a pitchfork was inserted after the drugs have taken effect. The worst part of a colonoscopy is the preparation. To view the inside of the intestines, they have to be cleansed. Otherwise, the view would be obstructed by feces, which could hide a pathological condition.

The four liters of liquid required as part of a colonoscopy bowel prep is euphemistically called GoLytely. But the intent is to literally flush out the bowels, enabling feces-free visual inspection. The night before the day of the test, patients are instructed to imbibe vast quantities of GoLytely until it comes out the other end crystal clear.

The electrician had a normal colonoscopy. A gastroscopy looks at the stomach and duodenum. It only takes a few hours for the stomach to empty itself of a meal, so the preparation involved is much less onerous. His gastroscopy was also normal. A CAT scan of the abdomen was normal.

Despite his pain, the investigations provided no clue. Was he a malingerer? Was this just another fictitious disorder? The surgeon was struck by the man's earnest personality and severe pain, so he arranged an exploratory laporotomy. A "quick look," a lap is a surgical procedure and the most invasive of tests for undiagnosed abdominal pain. Once the patient was anesthetized, the surgeon confidently cut him open. Staring out from the abdominal cavity were normal intra-abdominal organs. He felt around. A toothpick? A 10-year collective of chewing gum? A Barbie doll? Nothing. Everything was normal. He quickly sewed up his patient and decided the problem was functional.

That evening while finishing rounds, the surgeon reviewed some of the electrician's blood tests. Before choosing a career in surgery, he had dabbled in general internal medicine. As he reviewed the labs, he let out an audible gasp of glee. A routine blood count showed basophilic stippling of the red blood cells. When blood cells are reviewed under the microscope, the blood film is stained, to improve the diagnostic accuracy of the test. In basophilic stippling, dark blue granules dot the red blood cell when stained with "brilliant cresyl blue." They are observed in few conditions, one of which is lead poisoning.

The surgeon rushed to the bedside of his recovering patient, who hours before had been needlessly sliced open.

He questioned him about lead exposure. The only tantalizing hint was the electrician's 10-year habit of chewing three feet of electrical cable per day in lieu of cigarettes, a habit he had given up at age 39. He enjoyed the sweet taste of the plastic insulation wrapped around the cable. He had been warned about his habit by construction site managers, without an explanation.

The cable was tested for lead, which is added to ensure adequate cable flexibility. High levels were detected. His blood levels of lead were three times higher than accepted by occupational safety organizations. He was started on chelation treatment. EDTA was infused daily until blood lead levels dropped to undetectable values. Even though chelation is touted as a cardiac cure all, it only benefits the pseudo-doctors in white coats advising the treatment. In lead poisoning, however, it is the definitive treatment to bind the lead, followed by urinary excretion.

Lead was used in paints until banned in 1978. It was phased out of gasoline in 1995. Only about 10 percent of ingested lead is absorbed into the body of an adult, but up to 75 percent may be absorbed by a child. When it contacts the skin, only one percent is absorbed. About half of inhaled lead particles stay in the body. Most of the absorbed lead finds a home in bones, and it takes 30 years for a person to excrete half of their bone-based lead. Lead interferes with nervous system function, and is associated with lower I.Q. measurements.

When told of the dangers of his cable chewing habit, the electrician returned to cigarette smoking.

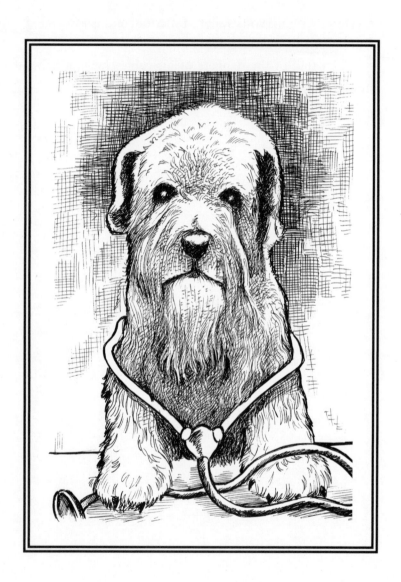

PROPER WOUND CARE

A 75-year-old woman finally underwent elective knee replacement. Plagued by years of osteoarthritis, exacerbated by her generous girth, she languished for a year on the waiting list before finally reaching the top. The surgery was uncomplicated. The muscles and ligaments of the knee were separated from the joint to allow entry into the joint capsule. Her old creaking knee joint, a cavern of bald white bone and debris, was replaced by a collection of plastic and metal. The lower femur, upper tibia, and patella were replaced with a cemented bionic joint, guaranteed to last longer than the patient. After a one-week convalescence, she limped to a rehabilitation facility for further occupational and physical therapy.

A widow with no children, her neighbors and pet were her main support. Her dog Barker was cared for by the Ellis family, who lived across the street from her neat bungalow.

When it was time to return home, she had a little trouble navigating over the three concrete steps leading to the front door. She grabbed the black iron railing and hoisted herself to the threshold. Fumbling for her key, it dropped on the welcome mat. The taxi driver had long since sped off, grumbling at the small tip. It took a few minutes, but she finally swept up the key and carefully opened the door. A warm musty breeze greeted her.

Within minutes, Jenny Ellis, all of 11 years old, presented a shampooed and excited poodle to her owner.

"Barky!" she exclaimed. "Did you miss me girl?"

The excited licks and yelps answered.

"She's been doing great, Mrs. Duncan," said Jenny. "We've been walking her three times a day and I think she lost some weight. She likes people food, but mom and dad said not to feed her from the table."

"Thank-you so much dear. I'll be baking you my short-bread cookies," said Mrs. Duncan, as she threw a wad of corned beef to her pet. It was clear Barky's excitement was based on more than just her loss of companionship.

As the months passed, Barky and her owner got fatter. Mrs. Duncan found her knee to be increasingly painful. She tried to complete her exercises, but the incision got angrier and angrier. Finally, she could take no more. She called up the Ellises and, apologizing for her imposition, asked if they could take Barky back while she transported herself to hospital. Barky was an unhappy dog.

In the emergency department, the orthopedic surgeon did a cursory exam after two minutes of questions. Mrs. Duncan winced as he moved her joint around and probed the incision.

"Looks infected ma'am," he drawled. "I don't feel any crepitus and the range of motion is good. You're afebrile and your white count is normal so I don't think you've got any systemic sepsis, but I feel some loculated areas over the joint, so I'm gonna have to tap it."

"What?" she responded.

"I gotta stick a needle in it," he explained.

"Oh," was all she could say.

He draped the knee in gowns of green, and sterilized the exposed skin with dollops of rust colored betadine. Using a 25-gauge needle, the caliber of a pin, he injected the skin, raising small blebs of local anesthetic around the knee. Each movement of the plunger attached to the needle caused sharp stabs of pain, soon replaced by numbness.

He waited for the local anesthetic to take effect and, after a few minutes, inserted a considerably larger 18-gauge (the smaller the gauge, the larger the caliber) needle into the infected incision on her knee.

As he felt the needle "give," an indication it had entered a liquid, he pulled up the plunger. Foul, yellow pus filled the syringe. Almost 35 cc. were aspirated. Mrs. Duncan's knee felt immediately better, less tense.

"Looks infected ma'am. I'll send it to the micro lab, but it's probably a staph or strep infection. We need to wash out the wound, so I'm gonna have to open up the incision and irrigate it with sterile saline. Why don't you come in for a few days. With the infection right on top of your knee, I want to give you some antibiotics. We can send you home in a few days on oral meds," said the orthopedic surgeon.

"Well OK," she replied, "but I have to get in touch with my neighbors to care for my Barky."

She was admitted to a room occupied by three other post-operative patients: two hips and a knee. She mostly kept to herself, keeping her drab and tattered drape encircled around her bed.

Her knee was much better, and she awaited word from her doctor about possible discharge. The nurses weren't sure when he would be available. On the evening of the second day, the curtain was drawn and in walked her surgeon, flanked by a mass of white-coated doctors.

"This is Dr. Fong," he began, pointing to an older Chinese doctor. "He's an infectious disease expert."

"This can't be good," she thought.

"We found a very unusual organism infecting your operative wound," he continued. "It's called Pasteurella multilocida. Do you have any dogs or cats at home?"

"Just Barky," she replied sheepishly, intimidated by the gaggle of doctors surrounding her. "He's my toy poodle. What's it got to do with my knee?"

"Well ma'am," he continued, "this type of bug is found in dogs and cats, particularly in their mouths. I know this is a strange question, but has Barky been licking your wound?"

"I thought it would help," she replied defensively. "Barky seemed to like licking it so I figured it wouldn't do any harm."

"The antibiotics will help and you can go home tomorrow, but don't let Barky lick anymore ok?"

And with that, the surgeon and his entourage turned and left. After a week of thrice daily pills, her wound had healed. Barky licked her face instead.

Pasteurella multilocida infections are frequently recognized after dog bites. Some bacteria, such as this one, are not normally found in human beings. Perhaps it's simply pushed out as other bacteria fight for space in the body. Regardless, the ability of the microbiology lab to finger-print the bacteria pointed towards a non-human source of the organism, and allowed the doctors to direct strange, but appropriate questions to the patient.

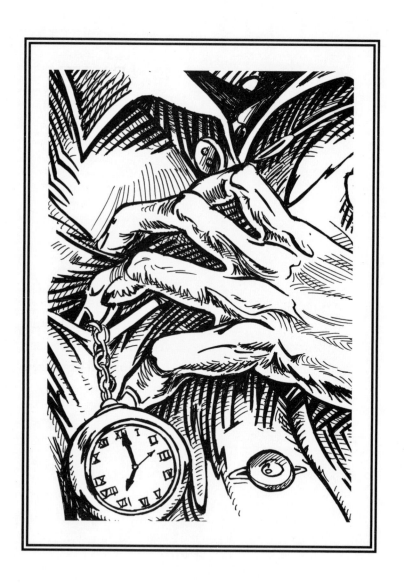

A TIMELY EVENT

A 62-year-old male physician, an emergency room doctor, was required by the hospital to upgrade his CPR (cardiopulmonary resuscitation) training. Recertification is necessary for license renewal every five years. The hospital organized CPR seminars for staff three or four times per year.

Joe was overweight, a smoker, and sedentary. The number of smoking physicians depends on the country in which they practice. French and Japanese doctors, for example, smoke much more than their North American counterparts. Joe was frequently seen around the perimeter of the hospital entrance with a cigarette in hand during lulls in the emergency room action.

Joe was very earnest and hard-working. He took less desirable night shifts to generate extra income. An intrinsic loner, he tried to engage the nursing staff with jokes and stories, but many found him uncomfortable to be with. A lifelong bachelor, he had a disheveled appearance. He always wore tattered sneakers, and bits of food hung from his full beard. He reeked of cigarette smoke, and his breath could be tear-inducing. Joe was unaware of his grooming difficulties. He strived to fit in, but like a gawky teenager, Joe didn't get it. He was an adequate emergency physician in a small city hospital.

He grumbled out of bed early on a Saturday morning and drove to the hospital auditorium. Joe wasn't feeling well, and wanted to get the whole thing over with. Nauseous and sweaty, he started practicing active resuscitation of the CPR doll.

"One, two, three, four, one, two, three, four," said Joe, pumping on the doll's chest as a colleague performed mouth to mouth.

The nausea continued and he began to sweat profusely. His gray hands were cool and clammy. Pressure slowly emanated from the center of his sternum, an expanding weight crushing his breath. His throat constricted, but he continued pumping the doll's chest, a half torso of plastic and rubber, vacant eyes transfixed on the ceiling.

"This is not happening to me," he rasped, denying the signs of the obvious. He had treated a hundred patients in his E.R. in the throes of heart attacks. Most lived, many died.

His partner stopped blowing into the doll's mouth. "Dr. Brittell, you don't look good. Have a seat, OK?"

Joe didn't hear the suggestion, his vision blurred, and he slumped forward grotesquely. As luck would have it, there were 50 qualified nurses and physicians within a 30-foot radius of Joe's collapse. Rushing forward, they quickly set CPR in motion. Hands pumping, ambu bags inhaling and exhaling. A stretcher carried Joe to the emergency room where his colleagues desperately tried to revive his shocked heart.

"BP is 80. Heart rate 130. He's in shock, someone hook him up to an EKG," the team leader calmly intoned.

Wires were connected to his chest, drenched in cold sweat. The electrical tracing confirmed the obvious: Joe was in the midst of a massive heart attack. A large portion of his heart was without blood flow and his body was shutting down. The weakened heart was unable to pump with enough force, and his organs were starving. Joe was rushed to the coronary angiogram lab where a hollow catheter was guided into his coronary artery, through which a balloon smashed open the blood clot.

Joe was saved, fortunate enough to have a massive coronary in an auditorium beside the emergency room amongst a roomful of nurses and doctors.

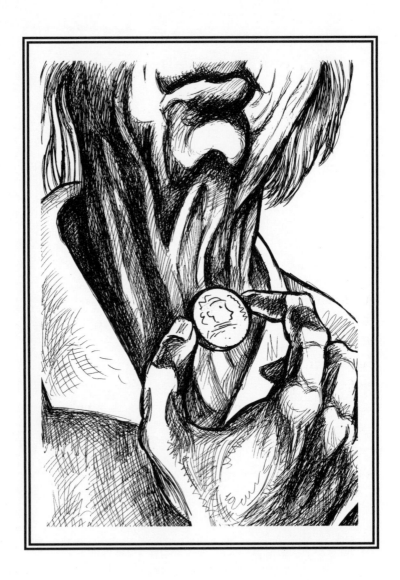

METAL ILLNESS

A disheveled 35-year-old man presented to hospital complaining of abdominal pain and asking for his stomach to be emptied. Reeking of urine, his clothes were drab, ragged, and stained. His long beard and mustache covered his face and lips. He had no known address, and periodically squatted in a tent city in a vacant industrial section of town.

On exam, he was thin with scrawny limbs and a protuberant abdomen. In no distress, he winced in pain as the doctor's hands moved across his swollen abdomen, especially in the left upper quadrant near his stomach. The vagrant had multiple hard masses that seemed to dart from beneath probing fingers.

"I think we should get a flat plate of his abdomen," the doctor called to the nurse, unsure what lay beneath the sallow skin and tissue. "There's something strange about this guy's stomach."

"I'm not doin' no x-ray!" howled the vagrant. "I jes want them things outta my belly."

The emergency physician was prepared to have the psychiatry service deal with the problem, but wanted to take a stab at explaining the enlarged belly.

"Maybe he has alcoholic liver disease," he thought. But the configuration of his abdomen was not typical for that condition. In alcoholics, impaired liver function leads to a condition called ascites, characterized by liters of straw colored fluid expanding the abdominal cavity. Up to 20 liters of ascitic fluid has been reported. Ascites causes smooth swelling, like a balloon, not the discrete lumps and bumps present in this man.

"Well, we won't know how to take them out unless we know exactly where they are," said the doctor, playing along with the mental illness. "An x-ray will guide us."

"I can tell you where they are, I was the one who put 'em in," responded the vagrant. "See here," he said, pointing to his lower abdomen, "these here scars are from me trying to get 'em out myself, but it pained me too much, so I want you to do it. That's what you get paid for."

"Just let me get an x-ray," pleaded the doctor, noting a collection of linear scars he had missed on first inspection.

The patient, perspiring and confused, said nothing else, which was interpreted as implicit consent. He was rolled into radiology, and moved to a flat narrow table. An x-ray plate was positioned beneath him. An x-ray machine swung over him and in less than a second, the test was complete. He immediately cried out in pain, holding his enlarged abdomen.

"That machine zapped me!" he bellowed. He sat up and took a swing at the unsuspecting technician, breaking her jaw with his clenched fist. He tried to leave the room, but before he could find the door, he fell to his knees. A code white was called and within seconds, two burly security guards easily subdued the struggling patient. He was tied to a bed, and the police were summoned for an anticipated assault charge. The technician became the next patient, and her swollen jaw was x-rayed, confirming that she would be drinking through a straw, and filing a grievance with her union and a long-term disability claim.

After the drama subsided, the doctor absent-mindedly reviewed the abdominal film, by now an afterthought. The police had requested medical clearance so that charges could be more conveniently filed at the division headquarters.

The doctor slipped the films into the viewing box and

was stunned by what he saw. Pliers, a small hammer, a zipper, pens (at least three), coins, wires, chain links — an enormous mass of metallic objects occupied the stomach, silhouettes struggling with each other to be recognized on the x-ray.

As the doctor appeared before the handcuffed patient, he briefly considered whether his charge would try to eat the handcuffs. "I see you have some unusual eating habits," he began. But he noticed something was amiss. The patient was sweaty and appeared more pale. He seemed short of breath.

"You zapped me with the rays, I'm gonna kill you," was the angry reply, as he struggled against the restraints. And with that, he collapsed, eyes and mouth wide open, vital signs absent.

A quick exam of his abdomen disclosed that it had suddenly become more distended. A code blue was called, fluids were infused, and CPR was initiated. Vital signs remained absent. After 45 desperate minutes, it was clear he was dead. The resuscitation was called off, and in its place a coroner was summoned. An autopsy was performed the next day.

Ninety-seven objects were fished out of his stomach and intestines. The cause of death was a perforation of the small intestine, the result of a sharpened Swiss Army knife, the price tag still dangling from a small metal circle at one end.

The intestinal walls have a withdrawal reflex. They shrink away from pressure, like a worm touched by a finger. This is why compulsive swallowers do not typically perforate their intestines. But the patient's gastrointestinal cavity was stretched so far by the collection of objects it could withdraw no further.

Among the retrieved objects were a pair of wire-rimmed glasses, various nuts, bolts, screws, and washers, $1.43 in coins, safety pins, nails, seven keys, a pair of nail clippers, a wristwatch, and a small belt buckle.

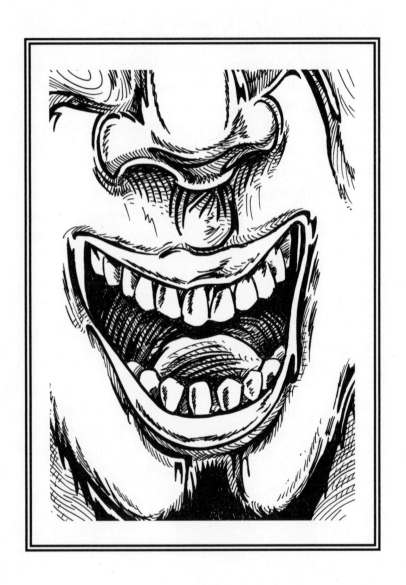

PERSISTENT
LAUGHTER

An 18-year-old presented to hospital after breathing in a small amount of insecticide, followed by nearly an hour of uncontrollable laughter.

An employee of a home and garden store, Ben had inhaled a single breath of concentrated insecticide. While preparing the concoction in the parking lot for application to the store's flowers, he inadvertently released the spray mechanism and deeply inhaled a concentrated burst of Bug B' Gone insecticide.

He immediately noted tingling of his fingers and toes followed by an enveloping sensation of giddiness and lightheadedness. Seconds later he began to guffaw uncontrollably. He recognized there was no reason for his burst of pathological and inappropriate laughter, but could not restrain himself.

The store manager, failing to see the humor and concerned about a visit from the workplace safety ministry, sent Ben to the hospital.

On exam, he was pleasant and his vital signs were entirely normal. Frequent loud bursts of laughter punctuated the history and physical. He could not suppress them, and his laughter echoed throughout the emergency room corridors. The staff found it unnerving.

"I just can't stop it Doc," he claimed. "I know there's nothing funny here but it just won't stop." This was followed by unrelenting high-pitched screams of apparent delight.

Scratching their heads, the emergency room staff had no idea how to handle this non-emergent problem. The neurologist on call was summoned. He too scratched his head, having never seen a case like this before. "Try some valium intravenously," he offered. "See if that calms him down."

By then, the laughter had persisted for nearly two hours. Ben's abdomen was beginning to bellyache.

As soon as 10 milligrams of intravenous valium were injected, the laughter ceased. A CAT scan of his brain revealed no masses or other abnormalities. Ben snoozed away the afternoon in a tiny enclosure of the emergency room. He had no recurrence, and found his laughter mechanism intact and appropriate.

Ben's emotional response, presumably in reaction to chemical exposure, is termed disinhibitory pathologic laughter. The first described case was the Joker of *Batman* fame.

There are a number of important anatomic areas in the brain involved in the generation and control of laughter, including the cerebral cortex, temporal lobes, hypothalamus, and bulbar nuclei. Laughter is regulated by a series of complex inhibitory stimuli. If these are interfered with in any way, persistent laughter may ensue, like a spinning wheel without a brake.

Epilepsy comes in many forms, including gelastic epilepsy, marked by uncontrolled laughter (*gelos* is the Greek term for mirth). Psychiatric disorders, various tumors, trauma, and a multitude of other neurologic conditions have been associated with pathologic merriment.

After excluding epilepsy, Ben's case was attributed to the insecticide. No other cases of persistent glee have been reported in the literature after insecticide poisoning. He was sent on his merry way and helpfully advised to avoid insecticide exposure.

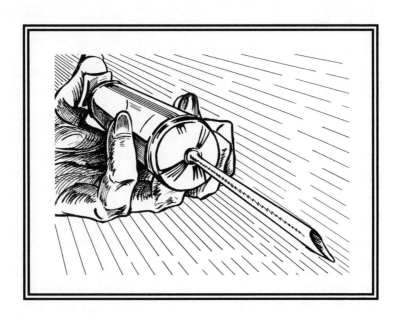

PERSISTENT ERECTION

An otherwise healthy 18-year-old boy presented to the emergency room with a persistent and painful erection (priapism) of 12 hours duration, unrelieved by ejaculation.

Sporting tented sweatpants and in obvious distress, he was whisked through triage by the sympathetic, smirking nursing staff. On exam, he was in obvious distress and uncooperative. His blood pressure was normal and he was tachycardic with a heart rate of 120.

"So when did this start?" asked the young emergency doctor, unable to avert her eyes from his erection.

"Can't I see a man?" he responded. "It's embarrassing

enough for me, you know. I don't need some chick looking at me and touching me down there."

"I'm the only doc on call," she said impatiently. "Now let's start again. When did this problem start?"

"Last night," was his brief morose reply.

"Any idea what caused it?" she inquired.

"If I knew I wouldn't be here," he said. "Look, it's killing me, can you give me something, or maybe do something?" he asked with a half smile.

Ignoring him, she proceeded to conduct an exam.

"Drop your pants," she ordered.

Reluctantly, his sweats fell to the ground, underwear to his knees. Staring at her was an erect, engorged member unhappily standing at attention. She felt like saluting and stifled her laughter. Priapism is a serious medical problem, she reminded herself.

"How long did you say it's been like this?" she asked, as she palpated his genitalia to ensure there were no other abnormalities.

"I told you, yesterday evening, about 12 hours," he replied, grimacing through clenched teeth. "It's really killing me and the damn thing is turning blue. I jacked off twice but the bloody thing doesn't seem to care."

"Masturbating doesn't help. It only makes it worse. Any

recent drug use?" she casually inquired, gently squeezing his testicles for abnormal masses.

He looked sheepish. "Like what?" he asked, one eye shut, his mouth in a rigid grin.

"You tell me," she responded.

"Well, I smoked some weed just before this all started, but I smoke a lot," he admitted.

"How much did you smoke?" she asked, transfixed on his foot-long erect member.

"I don't remember," he lied.

"OK, it doesn't matter," she said, "but if we don't get this thing down, you're going to have some serious trouble."

"Well how are you gonna get it back to normal?" he asked.

"We used to apply ice packs with ice water enemas, but we're more refined than that now," she replied. "We just need to perform corporeal aspiration and irrigation, and I'll need to do a few tests to confirm it was the pot that caused it," she added. "I have to call urology to sort this out." And with that, she turned and exited the room, leaving her patient wide-mouthed and frightened.

He waited another 15 minutes, his groin throbbing. Unfortunately for the young pothead, the urology resident was an attractive black-haired beauty.

"We're going to have to stick a needle in that," she explained, fondling him professionally. "It's called a priapism. Your blood went in, but it didn't come out, so I have to aspirate the blood from this area here," she said, pointing to the spongy swelling at the base of his penis.

"I'll give you some local anesthetic so it won't hurt. It's called a penile block," she said through her light blue surgical mask. Her eyes were beautiful and blue. He could see the expertly applied mascara above her mask. She was wearing tight black dress pants and a loose fitting white blouse that highlighted the curve of her breasts.

She prepped his penis with iodine and draped it in green towels so that only a small area was visible. She grasped his erect penis gently with gloved hands and stuck a needle at the base to anesthetize it from the effects of a larger needle. She waited a few minutes.

"Can you feel that?" she asked as she checked for sensation.

"Nope," came his tentative response.

"You might want to close your eyes at this part," she commented, "most guys do."

She took a large needle, punctured his penis, and drew back on the plunger. He watched the sludge of purple-hued blood fill the syringe as his erection gradually sagged. The urologist injected saline and aspirated further, repeating the procedure a half dozen times. Within 30 minutes his penis was back to its normal flaccid state.

"We need to observe you overnight. Lay off the pot, and this probably won't happen again," she intoned.

Priapism is the medical term for a painful unrelenting erection, without sexual desire, and unrelieved by ejaculation. It is named for the Greek god of fertility, Priapos. Causes include sickle cell disease, quadriplegia, certain medications, illicit drugs, leukemia, excessive alcohol use, and, surprisingly, excessive sexual activity.

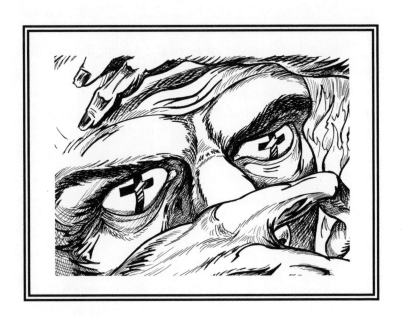

MISSING BODY
PARTS

A 27-year-old man was rushed to hospital. He was found by a pedestrian, lying in a downtown parking lot at 3 a.m. Blood-soaked and clutching a Bible with his right hand, his left hand and right foot were severed at the wrist and ankle, respectively. Protruding from his left eye was a serrated, wooden-handled, eight-inch steak knife. Right eye darting from side to side, he was mumbling incoherently.

After a rapid assessment by paramedics, tourniquets were tied to his limbs and he was bundled into an ambulance by two pairs of gloved hands. The knife was left in place, and the severed limbs were thrown into bags. Under the assumption that he was attacked by an unknown assailant, the police were summoned to the scene, and like dogs on a tree, yellow tape quickly demarcated a crime scene.

The man was assessed in the acute room of the emergency department. Blood pressure dangerously low, his veins were cannulated with two large-bore intravenous lines. Bag after bag of dark red blood was emptied through the IVs.

He was rushed to the operating room where his limbs were reattached. It was clear the eye could not be salvaged, and the enucleation that was initiated was completed by the ophthalmologist on call.

The following day he was questioned by police. Remorseful and with tears streaming down one cheek, he broke down and admitted his situation was the result of self-mutilation. He "auto-enucleated" his eye and performed a double auto-amputation. High on alcohol and amphetamines, and sleepless for days, he heard a voice from the Bible commanding him to cut off his limbs. He was prepared to sever his other foot, but lost consciousness from loss of blood before he could follow the instructions of his auditory hallucination.

Addicted to amphetamines for years, he became obsessed with Matthew 5:29; "If thy right eye offend thee, pluck it out and cast it from thee: for it is profitable for thee that one of thy body members should perish, and not that thy whole body should be cast into hell." High on drugs, he decided that the more body parts he could divest himself of, the purer he would become.

Acute amphetamine toxicity causes paranoia and agitation. Chronic amphetamine abuse often results in delusions and hallucinations, and has been associated with self-mutilaton. It may be difficult to distinguish the disordered thought process of chronic amphetamine abuse from schizophrenia.

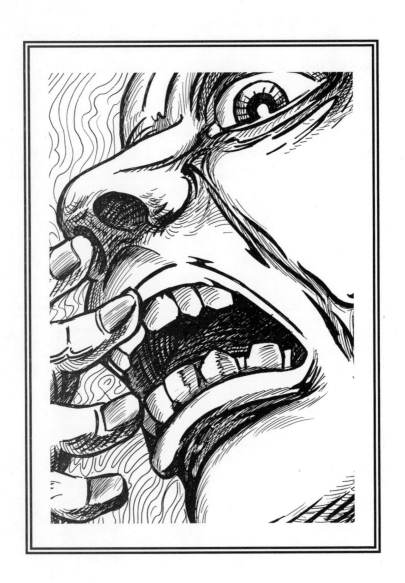

DEATH FROM BAD BREATH

A 20-year-old college student was delivered unconscious to the emergency room. His buddies reported that he was found in his room at noon after failing to make an appearance at breakfast or morning classes for two successive days. His worried friends broke down the door to his apartment and found him lying in bed seemingly asleep. Unable to rouse him, an ambulance was called.

There was no history of medical problems or hospitalizations. He was on no medications, to his friends' knowledge. Studious and earnest, he was not known to take illegal drugs or drink alcohol. There was no family history of serious medical issues. At the scene, the ambulance attendants did not find empty pill bottles, drug paraphernalia, or alcohol.

On admission, his coma was profound. His trachea was quickly intubated and he was placed on a ventilator to control his breathing. His blood pressure and heart rate were stable. He was hypothermic with a core body temperature of 34 Celsius (93 Fahrenheit). He responded to pain by withdrawing his limbs, but did not open his eyes in response to painful stimuli. His pupils were small and did not respond to light by constricting. A nasogastric tube was inserted from his nose into his stomach and activated charcoal was administered for a presumed drug overdose. The liquid black slurry was emptied into his stomach, creating a tar-like mess on his bed as huge gobs spilled over. A spontaneous brain hemorrhage was entertained; however a head CAT scan and spinal tap were normal.

A panel of blood tests was sent to the lab. A single startling abnormality was identified; his magnesium level was three times higher than normal, a finding that none of the doctors had ever seen before. They consulted online medical sites to assist in directing treatment. What was the cause of this surprising and bizarre finding? Hypermagnesemia in an otherwise healthy young man? There was only one possibility: ingestion, either accidental or deliberate.

He was treated with intravenous calcium and placed on emergent hemodialysis in an attempt to remove the excess magnesium from his blood as quickly as possible. During dialysis, his heart stopped. He was successfully resuscitated with atropine and a temporary transvenous pacemaker. Over the next four hours, he had relentless problems with abnormal heart rhythms and desperately low blood pressure. He was infused with four powerful intravenous medications simultaneously to try to raise his blood pressure to normal. Despite massive and heroic attempts at resuscitation, the medical team was unable to save his life, and within 12 hours of presenting to hospital he was declared dead.

Blood levels of magnesium are more often low than high. Elevated levels are a well-known result of over-indulgence in magnesium-containing laxatives, often administered in the hospital. This type of hypermagnesemia is called iatrogenic, from the Greek word *iatros* (meaning doctor). It may also occur from excessive ingestion of magnesium-containing antacids by misguided patients believing that if a little is good, a lot is better.

Puzzled doctors met with his distraught friends for further questioning.

"The only other thing I can think of was Ray's worry

about his bad breath," said his roommate Phil. "It became a bit of an obsession lately. He was always gargling."

With a list of magnesium-containing products in hand, the emergency room doctor asked if he knew what Ray was gargling with. "Epsom salts," was the reply.

Bingo. Epsom salts. Third on the list printed out by the troubled emergency doctor.

It was discovered that Ray was mixing boxes of Epsom salts with water and gargling. A month previously, Ray's girlfriend commented about his morning breath. High in magnesium, he was inadvertently, or perhaps intentionally, swallowing small amounts of this highly concentrated magnesium product with each gargle, leading to chronic magnesium intoxication.

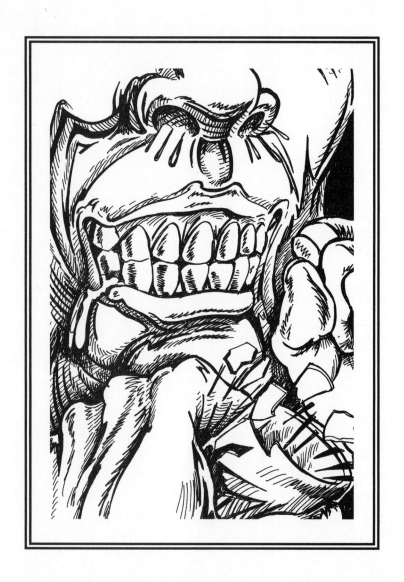

AN AGITATED BODYBUILDER

An agitated bodybuilder went to the office of his family doctor. Unable to sleep for three days, he demanded that his family physician attend to him.

"You'll have to wait your turn," said the nurse. "I don't care how big you are."

Scowling, his massive 5'7" 250-pound frame paced the length of the waiting room for an hour. The other patients shrunk away from him, fearful of his size. Recognizing the intimidation, and concerned by the potential explosiveness of the situation, the nurse directed him to an examining room. That helped little, as he was unable to sit still.

Wide-eyed and sweaty, he quickly got up from his

narrow chair beside the exam table, exited the room, and began to pace the hall. His ears were ringing.

"Arnold," greeted the doctor, "come on back into your room, I'll see you now."

Dr. Shimlin was a short and skinny man with a long nose. Hair surrounded his head in a half circle, with a central bald area. He wore thin wire glasses and spoke with a smile tattooed on his face.

"You look tense, Arnold. What's going on?"

Arnold spoke so quickly, it was difficult to understand him. His eyes shifted in every direction. While Dr. Shimlin sat in the narrow rectangular room, Arnold paced back and forth, brushing against the doctor's knees each time.

"I'm anxious, I need to get something to calm me down," Arnold said.

"What other symptoms are you having?" asked the concerned physician.

"You're a doctor, can't you see for yourself?" he yelled. He stood over the doctor, a menacing scowl on his face.

"Calm down, Arnold, I'm just trying to help," he said, wondering if he should continue the interview or call the police.

"All right. All right. Just listen damn it. I can't sleep, I'm bloody nervous. My stomach is doing butterflies. I feel like my heart is racing a mile a minute."

Dr. Shimlin noticed him biting his lower lip with his top teeth, drawing small swatches of blood. Diagnoses flew through his brain. Drugs? Steroids? Thyroid? Psychiatric? All of them?

"Have you been taking anything?" asked Dr. Shimlin.

"Just for the gym. I'm a bodybuilder obviously. How come you keep asking stupid questions?"

"What kind of stuff are we talking about, Arnold?" said the doctor.

"Just the goddamn caffeine tablets!" he screamed. "I've had enough of this shit. Give me something now!"

With that the doctor excused himself. Fearful of his safety, he asked his nurse to contact the police.

Within five minutes, two cops, a burly male and a slim female, appeared in the clinic. They were quickly briefed on the problem, and made their way down the hall, to find Arnold pacing.

"What seems to be the problem?" asked one of the cops.

"What the hell is it to you?" scowled Arnold. "Who the hell called you? I didn't do anything wrong." He tried to push through the narrow gauntlet of two cops and within 60 seconds was hog-tied, handcuffed, and restrained by the over-zealous couple.

In the police cell, Arnold continued pacing, screaming, and swearing. He vowed to track down the doctor, the nurse, and all of the staff at the clinic. Thinking he needed sedation and concerned that he would end up dead in his cell, the cops transported him to hospital.

"I can't figure out what the hell happened. One minute I'm talking to my former GP about caffeine tablets, and the next thing you know the cops are shoving me in the back of a cruiser."

"Tell me about these caffeine tablets," asked the gentle emergency room doctor of his shackled patient.

"There's nothing to them, I use them to improve my stamina. The more the better right?"

"Well how many do you use?" came the reply.

"More lately," he said.

"How many does more mean?" asked the doctor.

"About 25 tablets a day for the last five days."

The cause of this man's problems was obvious: he was suffering from the effects of acute caffeine intoxication. Each tablet, containing 150 milligrams of caffeine, was the equivalent of a strong cup of coffee. He was eating 25 before each workout, chasing them down with espressos. Instead of the usual 200 milligrams of caffeine a person might drink in a cup of coffee or tea, he was ingesting more than 4 grams in each of the last five days.

After discussion with poison control, he was treated as an inadvertent overdose. His stomach was pumped and filled with a slurry of activated charcoal to bind excess caffeine and prevent absorption. He was de-handcuffed and hospitalized for four days. He had evidence of muscle damage and kidney involvement on further testing of his blood, both of which returned to normal prior to his discharge from hospital.

Caffeine is absorbed very quickly from the stomach. Side effects include irritability, insomnia, nausea, diarrhea, and palpitations. Rarely, high dosages can result in seizures and coma. It is habit-forming, and abrupt cessation after regular use is associated with withdrawal effects including headaches.

Caffeine is an "ergogenic aid," meaning it improves performance. Although there is little evidence that the higher the dose, the better the performance, only very high doses are associated with any measurable improvement in physical performance. Caffeine is classified as a central nervous system stimulant and is frequently used by athletes. It is considered a banned drug by the International Olympic Committee, but low levels are accepted due to its nearly ubiquitous presence in foods and beverages. It would take at least six cups of concentrated coffee to run into trouble with the drug hounds at the Olympics, but you could probably absolve yourself of punishment by hiring a lawyer and claiming you had no idea how the caffeine (or anabolic steroid) found its way into your system.

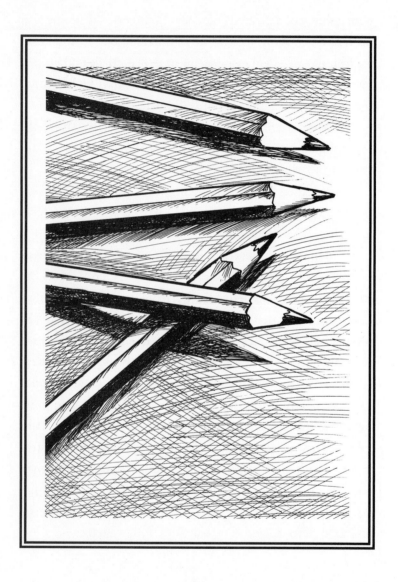

PENCIL PROBLEM

A 41-year-old body was discovered in a boarding house. Kenny was a long-time denizen of the hostel. Single and unemployed, he supplemented monthly government handouts by selling pencils to scrape by. His life was nondescript, his death, as the coroner discovered, less so.

On the streets as a teenager, he had worked in menial jobs for years before abandoning his remaining thread of pride and embracing government dependency. Kenny was popular with the other outcasts that inhabited the rundown neighborhood. He was not known as an alcoholic or drug addict. His behavior was invariably meek and polite, and he chose to mingle sparingly on the benches and corners. He never fought, yelled, cursed, or poked fun at others. In essence, Kenny was bland.

Dr. Hilroy was annoyed. Near the end of his week on call as the coroner, he had nearly escaped without being called on to do an autopsy. Aged and bothered by arthritis, he was tired of pathology and dreamed of retiring. Married and divorced over 40 years ago, he had never known his son, born soon after he had left his first wife. Dr. Hilroy didn't really care. He lived modestly with his third wife, and was never able to make enough money to graduate from his small bungalow to a condo. He supplemented his income as a pathologist at a small community hospital by taking government work as a local coroner. It paid reasonably well, but he was bitter that moonlighting was a part of his 70-year-old life.

"I should have been a surgeon," he muttered, as his scalpel sliced through Kenny's yellow skin. The corpse had a similar build to the doctor, same blue eyes and thin mouth. He peeled back the scalp. No evidence of head trauma. Using a compact and powerful circular saw, he sliced through the top of Kenny's head like the end of a loaf of bread. The brain tissue was the consistency of toothpaste. He removed the brain and sliced through it like deli meat. No bleeding.

"Must be his heart," he thought, as he moved on to the

thoracic cavity. His assistant split the chest and peeled back the ribs with a sickening crack. Dr. Hilroy cut out the heart, the size of his fist. Surrounded by normal amounts of oily fat, the heart reminded him to pick up a roast for evening dinner. He inspected the organ and its vessels, but there was no evidence of disease. He didn't care that he had not yet identified a cause of death. As a younger man, he would have been intrigued by this case, but his interest had died decades ago. Detached and sullen, he didn't care about this body, the case, or life. He wanted to go home.

"Just another dead, homeless alcoholic," he thought as he opened the abdominal cavity. Its putrid contents spilled onto the stainless steel table. Feces and blood mixed with chemical preservatives of the basement morgue.

The cause of death poked out towards him. Kenny's abdomen was filled with blood and a yellow pencil was embedded in his intestines, lead tip directed skywards. Further inspection disclosed a hole in his bladder. Kenny had inserted a pencil into his penis, which perforated his bladder, settled into his abdomen and caused a bacterial infection, peritonitis. Another case of autoerotic death.

Hilroy dictated a brief report and headed to pick up a roast. He never discovered who Kenny was, and never thought about him again from the moment he slipped off his dirty gloves.

If it fits into an orifice (ears, nose, mouth, vagina, rectum), it has probably been placed there. A famous abdominal x-ray shows an unopened umbrella. It was removed surgically for fear of inadvertently tripping the mechanism.

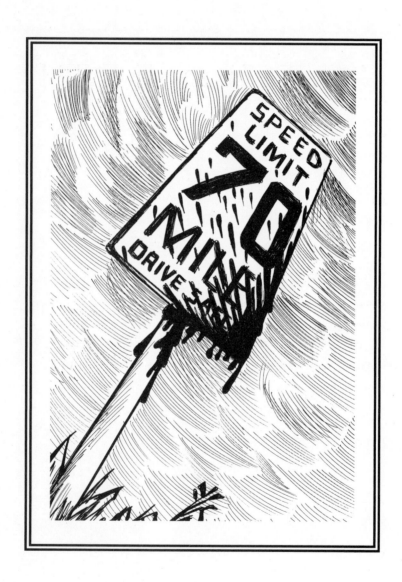

ROAD SIGN DEATH

The accident had occurred the previous evening. As the sun rose over the narrow two-lane country highway, a man was discovered cut in half, body parts separated by about 50 yards of asphalt. A trail of body fluids connected the two pieces in death. Splotches of blood, and bite-sized pieces of organs zigzagged toward the car. Police were summoned by a trucker, who hadn't stopped to provide further narrative. They halted what little traffic crept along the highway, and cordoned off the site with yellow plastic tape and neon orange pylons.

"Think it's that missing guy?"asked Williams.

"Obviously," replied his partner, sipping coffee from a styrofoam cup.

The victim's wallet, neatly tucked in the back pocket of his faded blue jeans, identified him as 38-year-old Jeb Macca. The cops knew him. His wife had reported him missing the previous day. He had argued with her about the money he didn't have that she was spending. Drunk, depressed, unemployed, and frustrated, he sped off in his BMW as the sun was setting. The accident scene was a good 80 miles from his house.

The lower half of Jeb's body, his pelvis and legs, was sitting in a two-door late model 3-series BMW. The floor of the driver's seat was dotted with purple clots of blood. Detective Hanson didn't think much about the fact he was removing a wallet from a body with no head and no torso. He wasn't sure how he was going to piece this together, but he was already certain it wasn't a homicide.

Up the road, Hanson's partner tended to the upper half of Jeb's body. It lay in a ditch, entrails hanging like wires from half a robot. Jeb's face was grey and twisted. He had bits of mud and grass coming from his mouth. Above him was a signpost advising travelers to obey the 70-mile speed limit. The numbers and letters on the sign were black. The sign's white background was sprayed with a thin film of Jeb's blood. The sign was about eight feet tall. Tissue hung from the rusted edges of the steel post.

"You thinking what I'm thinking?" said Hanson.

"Sure is an odd way to kill yourself," Williams replied. "What are we going to tell his wife?"

"It's not exactly something we can hide from her, unless it's a closed casket, or an open one with a blanket. We could always get the funeral home to sew him back together again. Maybe we should enlist all the king's horses and all the king's men," he joked.

The coroner examined the scene, and a tow truck loaded the car. The cleanup crews arrived later to remove both halves of the body.

Hanson began filling out his report. "The deceased was found along Highway 11. The upper half of his body was located in a ditch, and the lower half remained in the car, where it came to rest up the road 55 yards away. Based on the available forensics, it appears the decedent committed suicide by speeding down the highway at approximately 80 miles an hour. He appears to have turned his car in towards the sign and stuck his upper body out the window as the car passed the sign. He used it to sever his body in half."

"Why couldn't he just have taken pills like everyone else?" he wondered. He turned back towards town to break the news to the new widow.

AUTHOR'S NOTE

The medical cases in this book are based on fact, not fiction, and have been acquired from numerous sources. While some are based on conversations with colleagues, the majority come from leading medical journals, including *Lancet, Journal of Emergency Medicine, Journal of Accident and Emergency Medicine, Chest, Annals of Emergency Medicine, Journal of Nervous and Mental Diseases, Injury, Journal of Clinical Psychiatry, Journal of Trauma, Southern Medical Journal, British Medical Journal, Journal of the Royal Society of Medicine, Archives of Internal Medicine, Mayo Clinic Proceedings, General Hospital Psychiatry, International Journal of Care of the Injured, Annals of Allergy,* and the *American Journal for Medical Pathology.*